T0229295

Global Hand Surgery: Learning and Contributing in Low- and Middle-Income Countries

Editor

KEVIN C. CHUNG

HAND CLINICS

www.hand.theclinics.com

Consulting Editor
KEVIN C. CHUNG

November 2019 • Volume 35 • Number 4

ELSEVIER

1600 John F. Kennedy Boulevard ● Suite 1800 ● Philadelphia, Pennsylvania, 19103-2899

http://www.theclinics.com

HAND CLINICS Volume 35, Number 4
November 2019 ISSN 0749-0712, ISBN-13: 978-0-323-70900-2

Editor: Lauren Boyle
Developmental Editor: Kristen Helm

Hand Clinics (ISSN 0749-0712) is published quarterly by Elsevier Inc., 360 Park Avenue South, New York, NY 10010-1710. Months of publication are February, May, August, and November. Business and Editorial Offices: 1600 John F. Kennedy Blvd., Ste. 1800, Philadelphia, PA 19103-2899. Customer Service Office: 3251 Riverport Lane, Maryland Heights, MO 63043. Periodicals postage paid at New York, NY and at additional mailing offices. Subscription price is $435.00 per year (domestic individuals), $813.00 per year (domestic institutions), $100.00 per year (domestic students/residents), $501.00 per year (Canadian individuals), $947.00 per year (Canadian institutions), $546.00 per year (international individuals), $947.00 per year (international institutions), and $256.00 per year (international and Canadian students/residents). Foreign air speed delivery is included in all *Clinics* subscription prices. All prices are subject to change without notice. **POSTMASTER:** Send address changes to *Hand Clinics*, Elsevier Health Sciences Division, Subscription Customer Service, 3251 Riverport Lane, Maryland Heights, MO 63043. Customer Service (orders, claims, online, change of address): Elsevier Health Sciences Division, Subscription **Customer Service, 3251 Riverport Lane, Maryland Heights, MO 63043. Tel: 1-800-654-2452 (U.S. and Canada); 314-447-8871 (outside U.S. and Canada). Fax: 314-447-8029. E-mail: journalscustomerservice-usa@elsevier.com (for print support); journalsonlinesupport-usa@elsevier.com (for online support).**

Reprints. For copies of 100 or more of articles in this publication, please contact the Commercial Reprints Department, Elsevier Inc., 360 Park Avenue South, New York, New York 10010-1710. Tel.: 212-633-3874; Fax: 212-633-3820; E-mail: reprints@elsevier.com.

Hand Clinics is covered in *MEDLINE/PubMed (Index Medicus), Current Contents/Clinical Medicine, EMBASE/Excerpta Medica,* and *ISI/BIOMED.*

Contributors

CONSULTING EDITOR

KEVIN C. CHUNG, MD, MS
Charles B. G. de Nancrede Professor of
Surgery, Professor of Plastic Surgery and
Orthopaedic Surgery, Chief of Hand Surgery,
Michigan Medicine, Assistant Dean for Faculty
Affairs, Associate Director of Global REACH
University of Michigan Medical School, Ann
Arbor, Michigan, USA

EDITOR

KEVIN C. CHUNG, MD, MS
Charles B. G. de Nancrede Professor of
Surgery, Professor of Plastic Surgery and
Orthopaedic Surgery, Chief of Hand Surgery,
Michigan Medicine, Assistant Dean for Faculty
Affairs, Associate Director of Global REACH
University of Michigan Medical School, Ann
Arbor, Michigan, USA

AUTHORS

JOSHUA ABZUG, MD
Associate Professor, Departments of
Orthopedics and Pediatrics, University of
Maryland School of Medicine, Timonium,
Maryland, USA

NNENAYA AGOCHUKWU-MMONU, MD, MS
Clinical Lecturer, Department of Urology,
University of Michigan Medical School,
University of Michigan, Ann Arbor, Michigan,
USA; Department of Urology, University of
California, San Francisco, San Francisco,
California, USA

VINCENT ATIVOR, MD
Komfo Anokye Teaching Hospital,
Kumasi, Ghana

BRITTANY J. BEHAR, MD
Hospital of the University of Pennsylvania,
Philadelphia, Pennsylvania, USA

JAMES CHANG, MD
Department of Surgery, Chief, Division of
Plastic and Reconstructive Surgery, Stanford
University Medical Center, Stanford, California,
USA

KATHLEEN CHANG
Undergraduate Student, Stanford University,
Stanford, California, USA

KEVIN C. CHUNG, MD, MS
Charles B. G. de Nancrede Professor of
Surgery, Professor of Plastic Surgery and
Orthopaedic Surgery, Chief of Hand Surgery,
Michigan Medicine, Assistant Dean for Faculty
Affairs, Associate Director of Global REACH
University of Michigan Medical School, Ann
Arbor, Michigan, USA

OHENEBA OWUSU DANSO, MD
Komfo Anokye Teaching Hospital, Kumasi,
Ghana

PETER DEPTULA, MD
Resident, Department of Surgery, Division of Plastic and Reconstructive Surgery, Stanford University Medical Center, Stanford, California, USA

GEORGE S.M. DYER, MD
Brigham and Women's Hospital, Massachusetts General Hospital, Associate Professor of Orthopaedic Surgery, Harvard Medical School, Boston, Massachusetts, USA

KATE ELZINGA, MD
Clinical Lecturer, Section of Plastic Surgery, University of Calgary, South Health Campus, Calgary, Alberta, Canada

BOUTROS FARHAT, MD
Komfo Anokye Teaching Hospital, Kumasi, Ghana

MICHELLE A. JAMES, MD
Chief of Orthopaedic Surgery, Shriners Hospital for Children Northern California, Professor of Clinical Orthopaedic Surgery, University of California, Davis School of Medicine, Sacramento, California, USA

SCOTT H. KOZIN, MD
Team Leader – Touching Hands Project, ASSH, Chief of Staff, Shriners Hospitals for Children–Philadelphia, Professor of Orthopaedics, Lewis Katz School of Medicine, Temple University, Adjunct Clinical Professor of Orthopaedic Surgery, Sidney Kimmel Medical College of Thomas Jefferson University, Philadelphia, Pennsylvania, USA

DONALD H. LALONDE, MD
Professional Corporation, Dalhousie University, Saint John, New Brunswick, Canada

FRASER J. LEVERSEDGE, MD
Associate Professor of Orthopaedic Surgery, Adjunct Professor of Surgery, Plastic Surgery, Duke University, Durham, North Carolina, USA; Team Leader, Touching Hands Project, San

Pedro Sula, Honduras; American Foundation for Surgery of the Hand, Chicago, Illinois, USA

TERRY R. LIGHT, MD
Professor, Department of Orthopaedic Surgery, Loyola Stritch School of Medicine, Maywood, Illinois, USA

JACOB S. NASSER, BS
Clinical Research Associate, Department of Surgery, Section of Plastic Surgery, University of Michigan Medical School, Ann Arbor, Michigan, USA

MICHAEL T. NOLTE, MD
Resident Physician, Department of Orthopaedic Surgery, Rush University Medical Center, Chicago, Illinois, USA

KRISHNAN RAGHAVENDRAN, MBBS
Professor, Department of Surgery, University of Michigan, Ann Arbor, Michigan, USA

KAVITHA RANGANATHAN, MD
Resident, Department of Surgery, University of Michigan, Ann Arbor, Michigan, USA

JEANNE RIGGS, BS, OTRL, CHT
Clinical Specialist in Occupational Therapy, Department of Physical Medicine and Rehabilitation, Michigan Medicine, Ann Arbor, Michigan, USA

MARCO RIZZO, MD
Professor, Department of Orthopedic Surgery, Chair, Division of Hand Surgery, Mayo Clinic, Rochester, Minnesota, USA

SARAH E. SASOR, MD
Assistant Professor, Department of Plastic Surgery, Medical College of Wisconsin, Milwaukee, Wisconsin, USA

ANDY F. ZHU, MD
Hand Surgery Fellow, Department of Orthopaedic Surgery, Loyola University Medical Center, Loyola University Health System, Maywood, Illinois, USA

Contents

> The surgical burden of disease disproportionately affects individuals living in the developing world. In response, the surgical community has increased efforts to provide care to patients in these countries during short-term surgical trips. This article (1) summarizes the current concepts used in the economic evaluation of surgical outreach and (2) presents a conceptual model to describe the ideal approach to performing an economic analysis of surgical interventions in developing countries. This model may ensure that policymakers are provided with information to decrease cost and improve the access to specialty surgery in the developing world.

> The development of sustainable surgical systems in low- and middle-income countries is imperative given the rising burden of surgical disease processes. Surgical conditions now account for more than 11% of the overall burden of disease. Although the administration of surgical care has historically taken a variety of forms, a sustainable surgical model requires the utilization of robust clinical infrastructure, curricula for educating future staff and trainees, and research to promote quality improvement. Increasing the number of trained anesthesia providers, surgeons, and nurses is of utmost importance; task shifting may be necessary to most efficiently offset the shortage of health care providers.

> There is a growing need for surgical treatment of hand injuries in low- and middle-income countries (LMICs). This rise in disease burden places more pressure on these health care systems that are already struggling to provide access to surgical care for their patients. Hand surgery outreach initiatives have increased in recent years and provide much needed care and relief to these countries. There are significant patient-, physician-, institution-, and infrastructure-related barriers associated with developing an outreach initiative. Understanding these barriers is essential in establishing a successful and meaningful outreach initiative.

> The prevention and treatment of hand injuries in low- to middle-income countries needs to be a priority. Surgical outreach trips are a primary avenue for patients to

receive interventions. Challenges include language and cultural barriers, poor infrastructure, and limitations in a patient's ability to follow-up. Strategies to maximize patient functional outcomes include cultural competence, patient education resources, overcoming communication barriers, and using task-shifting strategies. Local therapists' knowledge and clinical skills can be enhanced. With improvements in data collection, therapists may contribute to gaining knowledge of outcomes in low- to middle-income countries.

The development of surgical capacity in the developing world is essential to address the global burden of surgical disease. Training local surgeons in low-income and middle-income countries is critical in this endeavor. The challenges to teaching hand surgery in the developing world include a shortage of local faculty, absence of a defined curriculum, no competency-based evaluation systems, few subspecialty training opportunities, and lack of financial support. To teach hand surgery in the developing world effectively, the authors suggest principles and components of a global training curriculum.

As the population increases in the world's poorest countries, the need for surgical interventions will increase. Short-term surgical missions can play an important role in increasing access to solve this disparity by providing much-needed surgical services to vulnerable populations in low-income and middle-income countries. As short-term surgical missions increase, it is important that basic ethical principles are a foundation in service delivery. By following ethical principles outlined in this article, abiding by common moral language, and establishing long-term relationships, a significant contribution can be made to global surgery to increase access and deliver high-quality surgery.

Hand surgery does not have to be expensive. Substituting evidence-based field sterility for main operating room sterility and using wide-awake, local anesthesia, no tourniquet (WALANT) surgery instead of sedation makes hand surgery much more affordable worldwide. This article explains how North Americans collaborated with Ghanaian hand surgeons and therapists to establish more affordable hand care in Kumasi. It describes how multiple nonprofit organizations collaborate to create transAtlantic Webinars and a reverse fellowship program to share hand surgery and therapy knowledge between North American and Ghanaian hand care providers.

Carefully planned, long-term partnerships can build surgical capacity in developing countries, which can save lives and alleviate suffering. Good partnerships are built around the goal of educating local staff. They involve consistent engagement with the same local hosts over time. Teaching is directed more broadly than just to surgeons; anesthesia, nursing, sterile processing, and biomedical engineering are also important partners.

Even in the most affluent country in the world there are many underserved population groups with limited or no access to health care. This article shares my experience with hand surgery volunteering with the Indian health service at Gallup, New Mexico and Chinle, Arizona. Although it has nuances with respect to logistics and challenges with regard to resources, the rewards of helping the patients in need has been among the best experiences of my career. I encourage anyone to consider domestic outreach because it reminds us of why we went to medical school.

Global outreach in hand surgery can be exceptionally rewarding for volunteers and their organizations, patients and their communities, and the host medical community. Success can be defined by individual cases that restore function and provide opportunities for a patient and family to contribute to society; however, the broader missions of medical collaboration, education, cultural exchange, and personal growth are critical factors toward building trust and establishing continuity of care for long-term success. Each outreach site and brigade encounters challenges; however, careful planning facilitates optimal conditions and reasonable expectations for enhancing outcomes.

Burns are devastating injuries that cause significant morbidity, emotional distress, and decreased quality of life. Advances in care have improved survival and functional outcomes; however, burns remain a major public health problem in developing countries. More than 95% of burns occur in low- and middle-income countries, where access to basic health care is limited. The upper extremity is involved in the majority of severe burn injuries. The purpose of this article is to review upper extremity burn epidemiology, risk factors, prevention strategies, and treatment options in resource-limited settings.

Although individual pediatric hand problems are rare, the combined burden of congenital anomalies, neuromuscular disease, and trauma is considerable in low-resource environments where treatment is unavailable. Surgeons from high-income countries respond to the need for care with short-term trips to low-resource environments to operate and teach local surgeons. Hand problems are amenable to this model, because they may be disabling and treatable with low-risk, low-resource surgery. Pediatric hand problems are especially compelling, because growth may adversely affect outcomes, and resulting disability is lifelong. This article addresses considerations for treating children's hands in low-resource environments, and approaches to specific conditions.

Hand trauma surgical treatment and perioperative therapy are often lacking in low- and middle-income countries resulting in high rates of patient morbidity following injury. Providing education through a multifaceted approach including in-person teaching, written resources, videos, and Internet and social media platforms and facilitating skill acquisition through simulation permits local providers to gain expertise in hand trauma care and thus benefits patients. This article outlines challenges faced by low- and middle-income countries in caring for hand trauma patients and possible implementable solutions.

Injury and musculoskeletal disorders are a major cause of death, disability, and decreased quality of life in developing countries. Thus, understanding the cost-effectiveness of orthopedic care in low- and middle-income countries may help to guide future outreach. A systematic review was conducted on the literature available on the cost-effectiveness of surgical trips that provided orthopedic-related care and extracted data regarding the cost-effectiveness of the orthopedic-related interventions. The cost-effectiveness of the interventions was determined using the WHO-CHOICE thresholds.

The Touching Hands Project was initiated as part of the American Society for Surgery of the Hand (ASSH) outreach effort in 2014. The project has expanded rapidly and has become a pillar along with education, research, clinical practice (patient care), and organizational excellence. This article explains the background behind The Touching Hands Project that leads to a groundswell of support for ASSH's commitment to outreach from the leadership, membership, and corporate members. The Touching Hands Project in collaboration with organizations with similar missions has greatly expanded hand care across the globe by focusing on education, patient care, surgery, and rehabilitation.

HAND CLINICS

SERIES OF RELATED INTEREST:

Clinics in Plastic Surgery
https://www.plasticsurgery.theclinics.com/

Orthopedic Clinics of North America
https://www.orthopedic.theclinics.com/

Physical Medicine and Rehabilitation Clinics of North America
https://www.pmr.theclinics.com/

THE CLINICS ARE AVAILABLE ONLINE!
Access your subscription at:
www.theclinics.com

Foreword

Learning and Contributing in Low- and Middle-Income Countries

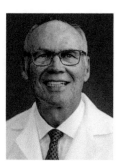

Joseph C. Kolars, MD

It is in your hands to create a better world for all who live in it.

—Nelson Mandela

This quote from a transformational leader on one of the continents at the epicenter of global health is no doubt metaphorical, but it evokes the issues that underlie a unique collection of articles for this issue of *Hand Clinics* devoted to Global Hand Surgery. First is the unique role the hand plays in culture and the human experience. Hands allow us "to do," turning thoughts into actions, unleashing our potential for productivity and creativity. Through movement and touch, our hands become conduits of expression, and the world understands and feels who we are. Uniquely human, the hand is often symbolic of our deepest connections to one another. When we "take a hand" in marriage, "lend a hand" to one in need, shake a hand in partnership, or raise a fist in protest, we are expressing sentiments that are germane to the human experience.

Second, our perspective on global health has been evolving. Earlier emphasis on "tropical medicine" and infectious diseases has given way to movements that advance health issues unique to at-risk populations, such as women and children. We've adopted a much more holistic understanding of health and how it relates to the 17 sustainable development goals outlined for all countries by the United Nations. Creating the ability for everyone to lead purposeful, meaningful lives is our over-arching goal, and we'd all agree that a good set of functional hands greatly enables this.

Of late, the global health movement is expanding its focus to include chronic diseases and trauma. The realization that in low-resource settings, more patients die from a lack of appropriate surgical care than from HIV, malaria, and TB combined is catalyzing momentum in surgery. "Outreach" has been a common way for surgeons to serve less privileged communities and address issues related to accessing care, but efforts directed at system strengthening, as frequently referenced in this collection of articles, are more likely to result in long-term sustainable changes. In light of its importance, those who focus on maximizing the function of our hands are crucial. People are more likely to do their best if they have good hands. Those who have devoted their careers to make this happen are to be applauded.

Joseph C. Kolars, MD
University of Michigan Medical School
6312D Medical Sciences Building 1
1301 Catherine Street SPC 5624
Ann Arbor, MI 48109-5624, USA

E-mail address:
jckolars@umich.edu

Hand Clin 35 (2019) xi
https://doi.org/10.1016/j.hcl.2019.07.003
0749-0712/19/© 2019 Published by Elsevier Inc.

hand.theclinics.com

Preface

Contribution of Hand Surgery for the Underserved and the Disadvantaged

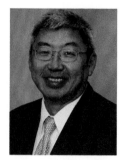

Kevin C. Chung, MD, MS
Editor

Hand Surgery has become a distinct specialty within medicine. Although Hand Surgery has a rich tradition in developed nations, the developing world is faced with an extraordinary burden in the care of hand injuries, diseases, and congenital problems that are often neglected. Hand surgeons are inherently altruistic, as shown by numerous volunteering trips led by hand surgeons in all regions of the world as well as in the Indian reserves and inner cities of the United States. To provide caring, educational, and ethical contributions, physician and surgeon volunteers require guidance from this global health issue, which provides "must-read" articles to facilitate productive programs. Furthermore, this issue shares reflective articles from surgeons whose lifelong devotion to volunteerism is presented in a first-hand accounting of personal experiences. When resources are limited for surgical activities, economic analyses of these efforts are critical to examine the best model for volunteering contribution by applying complex modeling exercises to justify the value of these volunteering efforts. In addition, we share the principles of cultural sensitivity and ethics that should serve as guiding principles for all involved. Serving in unfamiliar settings presents unique challenges. Several articles are devoted to impart tips to overcoming barriers for treating patients in resource-poor settings. A number of experts present their unique experiences in treating burns, congenital hand problems, and hand trauma in the developing world by highlighting novel, inexpensive treatment methods to adjust to the social and economic constraints by producing outcomes that are almost equal to those enjoyed by us in the developed countries.

I am grateful for the contributions by many of my colleagues, whose devotion to those in need is most inspiring. We are often mired in administrative headaches in our practices, but these volunteering trips reaffirm why we chose to be caregivers, for the singular purpose to do good. I would like to acknowledge the publishers of the *Hand Clinics* for giving us a forum to inform our collective experiences in guiding others to contribute in our own individual ways for making a better world.

Kevin C. Chung, MD, MS
Michigan Medicine
University of Michigan Medical School
1500 East Medical Center Drive
2130 Taubman Center, SPC 5340
Ann Arbor, MI 48109, USA

E-mail address:
kecchung@med.umich.edu

Hand Clin 35 (2019) xiii
https://doi.org/10.1016/j.hcl.2019.07.004
0749-0712/19/© 2019 Published by Elsevier Inc.

Economic Analyses of Surgical Trips to the Developing World
Current Concepts and Future Strategies

Jacob S. Nasser, BS, Kevin C. Chung, MD, MS*

KEYWORDS

- Economic analyses • Global surgery • Cost-effectiveness • Cost–benefit • Cost variation
- Developing world

KEY POINTS

- Current economic analyses of surgical trips are commonly nonstandardized cost-effectiveness analyses, therefore restricting policymakers from making proper comparisons of the health interventions.
- Standardized cost-effectiveness analyses need to be used in conjunction with cost–benefit analyses to provide policymakers with a more comprehensive representation of the health and economic impact.
- After the cost-effectiveness and cost–benefit analyses, research on predictors of cost variation must be performed to identify drivers of cost reduction for policy implementation.

INTRODUCTION

More than 4.8 billion individuals lack access to basic surgical care worldwide, most of whom live in low-income and middle-income countries (LMICs).[1] The lack of surgical care in LMICs is considered a neglected epidemic.[2] Before the 1990s, most global outreach efforts focused on providing medical care for communicable diseases such as human immunodeficiency virus–AIDS (HIV/AIDS), malaria, and tuberculosis.[3] Whereas approximately 3.83 million lives were lost in 2010 because of HIV/AIDS, malaria, and tuberculosis, a substantially greater number, 16.9 million lives, were lost because of insufficient surgical care in the same year.[4] Despite the outdated notion that surgery is too complex to be performed in a low-resource setting, global surgical outreach is becoming progressively recognized as an imperative element of global health development.[2,5]

Individuals with surgically amenable conditions face substantial economic challenges; 21 trillion dollars will be lost in economic output as a result of the surgical burden of disease from 2015 to 2030.[1] This loss of economic output is attributed to the barriers in access, availability, affordability,

Funding: The work was supported by a Midcareer Investigator Award in Patient-Oriented Research (2 K24-AR053120-06) to K.C. Chung. The content is solely the responsibility of the authors and does not necessarily represent the official views of the National Institutes of Health.
Funded by: National Institute of Arthritis and Musculoskeletal and Skin Diseases. Grant number(s): 2 K24-AR053120-06.
Disclosure Statement: The authors did not have any relationship with a commercial company with a financial interest in the subject discussed in this article.

Comprehensive Hand Center, Michigan Medicine, 1500 E. Medical Center Drive 2130 Taubman Center, SPC 5340, Ann Arbor, MI 48109-5340, USA
* Corresponding author.
E-mail address: kecchung@med.umich.edu

Hand Clin 35 (2019) 381–389
https://doi.org/10.1016/j.hcl.2019.06.001

hand.theclinics.com

and acceptability of surgical care in LMICs.[6] For example, some individuals are unable to access appropriate surgical specialists for treatment, resulting in severe disability or even death. The *Lancet* Commission on Global Surgery was established in 2014 to help combat the direct and indirect consequences of the surgical burden of disease.[7] The commission focuses on improving global health care delivery, education, economics, and management to address the gaps in safe and affordable surgical care.[1,8] The surgical community has since increased their outreach efforts to echo the mission of this organization.

Surgery in the developing world primarily consists of basic services for Caesarean sections, laparotomies, trauma management, and pediatric surgery.[9] Many of the conditions in LMICs require subspecialty surgical care. For instance, orthopedic surgeons are needed to help treat individuals with deformations of the musculoskeletal system due to severe trauma.[10] The surgical community uses a variety of ways to provide subspecialty surgical care to individuals living in LMICs, commonly through short-term surgical trips.[11] Evaluating the health and economic impacts of the surgical interventions performed during surgical outreach, using an assortment of analyses, is vital to the sustainability of these surgical outreach efforts.

Numerous economic analyses have been performed to evaluate the sustainability of particular surgical interventions in LMICs. This article (1) summarizes the current concepts used in the economic evaluation of surgical global outreach efforts and (2) identifies potential areas of improvement that may lead to the advancement of such evaluations. Furthermore, the authors created a conceptual model to describe the ideal approach for economic analyses of surgical trips in LMICs.

CURRENT CONCEPTS

The World Health Assembly declared surgical care a priority initiative in 2015, requesting the "awareness of cost-effective [surgical] options be made more apparent."[12] As a result, there have been extensive cost-effectiveness analyses examining the feasibility of specific surgical interventions in plastic surgery,[13–15] neurosurgery,[16] pediatric surgery,[17] and ophthalmology[18–20] as well as other subspecialties.[21–23] Despite suggestions that surgery is too expensive to be performed in LMICs,[24] research has shown some surgical interventions in LMICs may be cost-effective.[25] The current model focuses on conducting cost-effectiveness analyses to determine which surgical interventions should be prioritized in a resource-limited environment to make the greatest impact (**Fig. 1**).[26,27]

Cost-effectiveness analyses assess the costs and related benefits of a health intervention.[28,29] Common metrics for cost-effectiveness analyses include cost per quality-adjusted life years (QALYs) or cost per disability-adjusted life years (DALYs), both of which take into account the costs and benefits of averting mortality and morbidity.[30] When examining the health benefits of a surgical intervention performed in an LMIC, researchers usually report the cost-effectiveness in terms of cost per DALY-averted.[15,16,19,22] The cost per DALY-averted represents the cost, in monetary terms, required to avert 1 year of life that would otherwise be lost because of the morbidity and mortality of a particular surgical condition.[31,32]

The World Health Organization developed CHOosing Interventions that are Cost-Effective (WHO-CHOICE) methods to standardize cost-effectiveness analyses on global health interventions. WHO-CHOICE methods have requirements on describing the overall study design, estimating costs, approximating health effects, and discounting costs.[33,34] Nolte and colleagues[35] performed a systematic review of economic analyses of surgical trips to examine the adherence to this standardized criterion. The investigators concluded that none of the cost-effectiveness analyses in this review adhered to the WHO-CHOICE

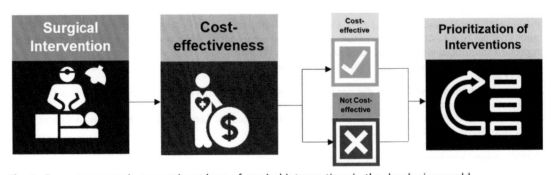

Fig. 1. Current concepts in economic analyses of surgical interventions in the developing world.

methods. If a standardized methodology is not used to report the findings of a cost-effectiveness analysis, then the implications of the investigations are questioned. Although some individuals have concluded that certain surgical interventions in the developing world are not cost-effective, it is not indicative that the intervention should be considered low priority or that intervention should not be performed in a low-resource setting. Rather, further, more detailed analyses are needed to determine (1) how the surgery can become more cost-effective and (2) how monetary support for interventions performed in LMICs can continue.

DEVELOPMENT OF ECONOMIC ANALYSES

Economic analyses must be used in conjunction with each other to have meaningful effects on the development of global surgery. **Table 1** provides a summary of the various economic analyses used to assess global health interventions. **Fig. 2** illustrates the ideal approach for economic analyses of surgical interventions in LMICs. If an intervention is not considered cost-effective, then further research is needed to determine potential drivers of cost variation. These predictors of cost variation can then be used to implement policy focused on reducing cost in that area of spending. Conversely, if an intervention is not considered cost-effective and no cost variation is identified, then prioritization decisions must be made.

In addition to cost-effectiveness analyses, cost–benefit analyses should be used to convey the economic benefit of particular health interventions on society.[36,37] Cost–benefit analyses differ from cost-effectiveness analyses by measuring both the costs and benefits of an intervention in monetary units. Conversely, cost-effectiveness

analyses use the amount of DALYs averted, or QALYs gained, to measure benefits. The results of a cost–benefit analysis can be used to decide which programs have the highest return on investment.[36,37] If the results of a cost–benefit analysis suggest that a net economic benefit exists, then a cost variation analysis is not needed. Conversely, if there is no net economic benefit, then a cost variation analysis may help improve the net economic benefit of the surgical interventions performed. Cost–benefit analyses, in conjunction with cost-effectiveness analyses, should be used to determine whether a cost variation analysis is warranted (**Fig. 3**).

Cost-Effectiveness Analyses

Researchers examining the cost-effectiveness of surgical trips to LMICs should adhere to standardized WHO-CHOICE methods.[30] The lack of adherence to a standard makes it difficult for policymakers to compare the effectiveness of different interventions. For example, various cost-effectiveness analyses lack similarity in their accounting methodology. Tadisina and colleagues[13] conducted a cost-effectiveness analysis of hand surgery performed during a surgical trip to Honduras. In this analysis, the investigators did not discount the costs of the surgical trip. Alternatively, Baltussen and colleagues[19] examined the cost-effectiveness of cataract surgery in developing countries and discounted the costs at an annual rate of 3%, as suggested by WHO-CHOICE methods. The 2 studies did not adhere to similar methods in their investigations: 1 study is overestimating the costs, whereas the other is underestimating the costs. Thus, it may be troublesome when the results of both studies are

---

Table 1
Economic analyses used to assess surgical interventions in the developing world

Type of Economic Analysis	Definition	Purpose	Metric Reported
Cost-effectiveness	An analysis used to assess the monetary cost and related health benefits of a particular surgical intervention	Define the cost of a particular health outcome	Cost per DALYs averted Cost per QALYs gained
Cost–benefit	An analysis used to measure both the costs and benefits of a surgical intervention in monetary units	Determine which health intervention has the highest return on investment	Dollars ($)
Cost Variation	An analysis used to identify whether high variance exists for a particular area of spending	Identify drivers of cost variation that can be used to reduce the cost of a particular area of spending	—

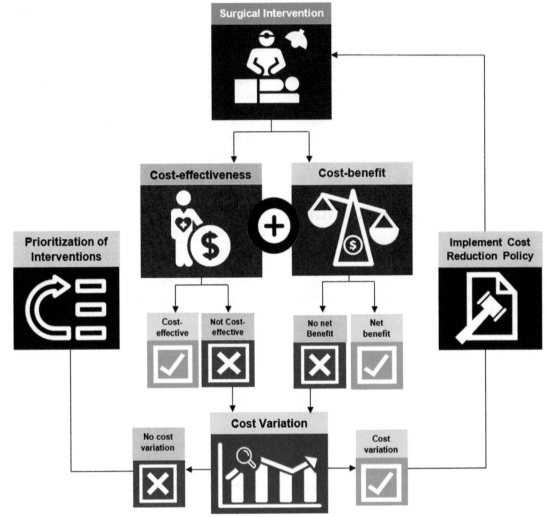

Fig. 2. Conceptual model for development of economic analyses of surgical interventions in the developing world.

used to implement policy regarding resource allocation.

Efforts to educate local providers in the developing world during short-term surgical trips have become increasingly common.[38–40] For example, ReSurge International performs visiting educator surgical trips, in which the traveling organization educates local surgeons on particular operations.[41] The impact of these trips usually occurs after the organization leaves the host country. To the best of the authors' knowledge, no methodology exists to evaluate the cost-effectiveness of such surgical trips. With an established methodology, policymakers would be able to better understand the economic impact of educating local physicians on treating surgical conditions.

The results of economic analyses are most meaningful when they are compared with other widely accepted interventions. Grimes and colleagues[18] determined that elective inguinal hernia repair surgery is considered cost-effective in LMICs by comparing the cost-effectiveness to accepted global health interventions, such as oral rehydration therapy or breast feeding promotion. This comparison helps provide evidence that both interventions are beneficial and require similar attention. Although cost-effectiveness analyses are of interest to decision-making bodies, cost–benefit analyses appeal to those providing funding and support of global surgery outreach efforts to LMICs.

Cost–Benefit Analyses

Cost–benefit analyses are used to determine the economic benefit of an intervention in monetary terms.[36,42] They are of interest to program

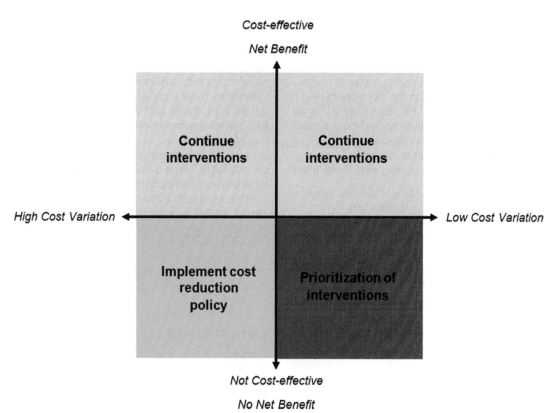

Fig. 3. Implementing policy based on cost variation analyses.

financiers because they demonstrate the value of an intervention using a simple metric (dollar). Although such analyses are of interest to decision-making bodies, there are few publications in global surgery literature.[43–45] This under-utilization is attributed to the difficulty of placing a monetary value on health benefits.[43,46]

To perform a cost–benefit analysis, one must

1. Determine the total cost of the surgical trip
2. Calculate the potential benefits of the health interventions
3. Convert the health benefits to monetary terms.

Researchers use different approaches to convert the potential health benefits of an intervention to a monetary value. These include the value of a statistical life year approach, in which value is placed on an individual's willingness to pay for a reduction in mortality risk; the human capital approach, in which value is placed on an individual's potential economic productivity; or the willingness-to-pay approach, in which value is placed on an individual's willingness to pay for certain health benefits.[37,43,47] The most common method used is the value of a statistical life year approach.[43,44,48,49]

A cost–benefit analysis of cleft lip and palate interventions was performed at a single center in Nepal to estimate the economic impact of cleft lip and cleft palate repair. Using the value of a statistical life approach, the net economic benefit at this single center was between $56,919 and $143,363 for cleft lip repair and between $152,372 and $375,412 for cleft palate repair.[44] The investigators concluded that cleft lip and cleft palate repairs performed at this center had a substantial impact on the economic health in Nepal. Calculation of the net economic benefit informs policymakers on the cost-saving impact each dollar spent on the program will have.

Cost Variation Analyses

Global health care spending is expected to increase from 9.2 trillion to 24.2 trillion dollars between 2014 and 2040.[50] Increases in the expenditures of US nonprofit and volunteer divisions have also been observed.[51] Policymakers are trying to develop different strategies that minimize discrepancy spending in hopes of providing high-quality and low-cost care to patients in LMICs. One strategy used to decrease spending in health care is determining variations in spending. In the United States, variations in hospital costs have been studied in various fields, including plastic,[52] general,[53] and cardiac surgery.[54] Similar analyses can be used to determine drivers for cost variation and increase the effectiveness of surgical trips in the developing world. Exploring various ways to reduce costs while conserving high-quality care should be a priority for surgical outreach organizations.

To perform a cost variation analysis of a surgical trip conducted in the developing world, one must

1. Calculate the difference between the incurred and expected cost of a surgical trip
2. Create a model to assess the link between possible predictors and total cost of the surgical trip
3. Perform a root cause analysis to determine the cause expenditure variation.

These predictors may include organization, number or profession of personnel needed on the surgical trip, and cost classifications (personnel, materials and supplies, donated materials), among others. In a cost variation analysis published by Harris and colleagues,[55] the investigators examined the cost of urethroplasty procedures. First, they developed a log cost linear regression model to determine which variables were associated with increased cost. Procedures with extreme cost, those in the top 20th percentile, were then identified using the same variables as for log cost. Finally, they compared the variables between the extreme cost category and increased procedural cost category to determine predictors of cost variation. When determining these predictors, the investigators controlled for patient age, race, and year using a multivariable analysis. Although this analysis did not examine cost variation of global outreach programs, the methods used may serve as a model for cost variation analyses of surgical trips to LMICs.

Cost variation analyses may help increase the cost-effectiveness and improve the overall net economic benefit of surgical interventions performed in LMICs (see **Fig. 3**). If surgical interventions performed in a surgical trip are considered cost-effective and a net economic benefit exists, then no cost variation analysis is warranted. Conversely, if an intervention is not considered cost-effective, or if no economic benefit is observed, then a cost variation analysis should be done to determine areas of spending that can be reduced to improve both the cost-effectiveness and overall economic benefit. For example, a hypothetical cost variation analysis may show that travel expenses for personnel are a predictor for increased cost. When performing a root cause analysis, policymakers determine that airfare for personnel is the reason for increased travel cost. Policymakers may then require that local volunteers are recruited during various surgical trips to help with trivial tasks, rather than flying out volunteers to help with the same responsibilities. Additionally, policymakers may strive to increase the economic impact by implementing programs that focus on educating local providers. This may permit local providers to perform the learned procedure on thousands of individuals and maximize the impact of the surgical trip. After implementation of such policy, cost-effectiveness and cost–benefit analyses must be performed to determine if the new policy reduced the surgical trip cost. Cost variation analyses may ensure that priority-setting decisions are only used as a last resort.

IMPLICATIONS OF ECONOMIC ANALYSES

Surgical care delivery in LMICs is hindered by the (1) lack of material resources, (2) inexperienced health care personnel, and (3) inefficient resource management strategies.[56–60] Economic analyses provide insight about the value of the surgical health interventions performed in the developing world.[17] Because of the resource-limited settings in the developing world, policymakers must determine which treatments should be prioritized and develop strategies to reduce the costs of interventions that are too costly to be performed in a resource-limited environment. These policymakers include government departments, nongovernmental organizations, individual or institutional decision-makers, private enterprises, consumers, and external donors.[61] Policymakers consider information on cost-effectiveness, economic benefit, medical suitability, and epidemiologic appropriateness when developing strategies used to guide global health development.[62,63] Understanding the economics of the various global surgery interventions are vital to the development of these efforts in LMICs.

SUMMARY

As the surgical burden of disease continues to grow, it becomes imperative to study the effectiveness of the interventions used to alleviate the burden. Health care resources in LMICs are limited, thus policy must be implemented to maximize the benefits of the interventions while minimizing the cost. Policymakers must focus on implementing cost reduction policies before making decisions regarding priority settings. A combination of cost-effectiveness, benefit, and variation analyses will provide policymakers with the appropriate information to develop the most effective policy. Each economic analysis provides different evidence, independently appealing to a different audience.

Moving forward, research on the economic value of surgery in the developing world must focus on standardized cost-effectiveness analyses in conjunction with cost–benefit and cost variation analyses. The development of a methodological standard for cost–benefit and cost variation analyses is also warranted, as it may increase the reliability of economic analyses. Additionally, more detailed data on cost and clinical outcomes of the interventions performed in the developing world will help promote additional research on the effectiveness and sustainability of such humanitarian outreach efforts.

REFERENCES

1. Alkire BC, Shrime MG, Dare AJ, et al. Global economic consequences of selected surgical diseases: a modelling study. Lancet Glob Health 2015; 3(Suppl 2):S21–7.
2. Grimes CE, Lane RHS. Surgery and the global health agenda. J R Soc Med 2013;106(7):256–8.
3. Shrime MG, Bickler SW, Alkire BC, et al. Global burden of surgical disease: an estimation from the provider perspective. Lancet Glob Health 2015;3: S8–9.
4. Rayne S, Burger S, Van Straten S, et al. Setting the research and implementation agenda for equitable access to surgical care in South Africa. BMJ Glob Health 2017;2(2):e000170.
5. Shawar YR, Shiffman J, Spiegel DA. Generation of political priority for global surgery: a qualitative policy analysis. Lancet Glob Health 2015;3(8):e487–95.
6. Ologunde R, Maruthappu M, Shanmugarajah K, et al. Surgical care in low and middle-income countries: Burden and barriers. Int J Surg 2014;12(8): 858–63.
7. The Commission Process 2015. Available at: https://www.lancetglobalsurgery.org/background. Accessed January 16, 2018.
8. Mukhopadhyay S, Ojomo K, Nyberger K, et al. Lancet commission on global surgery. Iran J Pediatr 2017;27(4):1–7.
9. Wright I, Walker I, Yacoub M. Specialist surgery in the developing world: luxury or necessity? Anaesthesia 2007;62(s1):84–9.
10. Brouillette MA, Kaiser SP, Konadu P, et al. Orthopedic surgery in the developing world: workforce and operative volumes in Ghana compared to those in the United States. World J Surg 2014;38(4):849–57.
11. Kynes JM, Zeigler L, McQueen K. Surgical outreach for children by international humanitarian organizations: a review. Children 2017;4(7):53.
12. Raykar N, Mukhopadhyay S, Ng-Kamstra JS, et al. Progress in achieving universal access to surgical care: an update and a path forward. Bull Am Coll Surg 2016;101(6):12–8.
13. Tadisina KK, Chopra K, Tangredi J, et al. Helping hands: a cost-effectiveness study of a humanitarian hand surgery mission. Plast Surg Int 2014;2014: 921625.
14. Hackenberg B, Ramos MS, Campbell A, et al. Measuring and comparing the cost-effectiveness of surgical care delivery in low-resource settings: cleft lip and palate as a model. J Craniofac Surg 2015;26(4):1121–5.
15. Hamze H, Mengiste A, Carter J. The impact and cost-effectiveness of the Amref Health Africa-Smile Train Cleft Lip and Palate Surgical Repair Programme in Eastern and Central Africa. Pan Afr Med J 2017;28:35.
16. Punchak M, Lazareff JA. Cost-effectiveness of short-term neurosurgical missions relative to other surgical specialties. Surg Neurol Int 2017;8:37.
17. Saxton AT, Poenaru D, Ozgediz D, et al. Economic analysis of children's surgical care in low- and middle-income countries: a systematic review and analysis. PLoS One 2016;11(10):e0165480.
18. Grimes CE, Henry JA, Maraka J, et al. Cost-effectiveness of surgery in low-and middle-income countries: a systematic review. World J Surg 2014;38(1): 252–63.
19. Baltussen R, Sylla M, Mariotti SP. Cost-effectiveness analysis of cataract surgery: a global and regional analysis. Bull World Health Organ 2004;82(5): 338–45.
20. Baltussen R, Smith A. Cost effectiveness of strategies to combat vision and hearing loss in sub-Saharan Africa and South East Asia: mathematical modelling study. BMJ 2012;344:e615.
21. Shrime MG, Sleemi A, Ravilla TD. Charitable platforms in global surgery: a systematic review of their effectiveness, cost-effectiveness, sustainability, and role training. World J Surg 2015;39(1):10–20.
22. Shillcutt SD, Clarke MG, Kingsnorth AN. Cost-effectiveness of groin hernia surgery in the Western Region of Ghana. Arch Surg 2010;145(10): 954–61.
23. Chen AT, Pedtke A, Kobs JK, et al. Volunteer orthopedic surgical trips in Nicaragua: a cost-effectiveness evaluation. World J Surg 2012; 36(12):2802–8.
24. Gosselin RA, Gyamfi Y-A, Contini S. Challenges of meeting surgical needs in the developing world. World J Surg 2011;35(2):258–61.

25. Marseille E, Morshed S. Essential surgery is cost effective in resource-poor countries. Lancet Glob Health 2014;2(6):e302–3.

26. Dare AJ, Lee KC, Bleicher J, et al. Prioritizing surgical care on national health agendas: a qualitative case study of Papua New Guinea, Uganda, and Sierra Leone. PLoS Med 2016;13(5):e1002023.

27. Tollefson TT, Larrabee WF. Global surgical initiatives to reduce the surgical burden of disease. JAMA 2012;307(7):667–8.

28. Weinstein MC, Stason WB. Foundations of cost-effectiveness analysis for health and medical practices. N Engl J Med 1977;296(13):716–21.

29. Robinson R. Cost-effectiveness analysis. BMJ 1993; 307(6907):793–5.

30. Edejer TT-T, Baltussen R, Adam T, et al. WHO guide to cost-effectiveness analysis. Geneva (Switzerland): World Health Organization; 2002.

31. Zarate V. DALYs and QALYs in developing countries. Health Aff 2007;26(4):1197–8.

32. Robberstad B. QALYs vs DALYs vs LYs gained: what are the differences, and what difference do they make for health care priority setting? Nor Epidemiol 2009;15(2):183–91.

33. Edejer TT-T. Making choices in health: WHO guide to cost-effectiveness analysis, vol. 1. Geneva (Switzerland): World Health Organization; 2003.

34. Johns B, Baltussen R, Hutubessy R. Programme costs in the economic evaluation of health interventions. Cost Eff Resour Alloc 2003;1(1):1.

35. Nolte MT, Maroukis BL, Chung KC, et al. A systematic review of economic analysis of surgical mission trips using the World Health Organization criteria. World J Surg 2016;40(8):1874–84.

36. Robinson R. Cost-benefit analysis. BMJ 1993; 307(6909):924–6.

37. Edwards C. Social cost-benefit analysis–the available evidence on drinking water. Pond, K, Pedley, S, Edwards, C,(2008) Valuing water–valuing wellbeing: a guide to understanding the costs and benefits of water interventions. Geneva (Switzerland): World Health Organization; 2008. p. 1–23. Available at: http://www who int/water_sanitation_health/economic/cb_interventions/en/index html. Accessed April 29, 2011. 2008.

38. McCullough M, Campbell A, Siu A, et al. Competency-based education in low resource settings: development of a novel surgical training program. World J Surg 2018;42(3):646–51.

39. Yang GP, Wren SM. Enhancing local resources in low- and middle-income countries through education. JAMA Surg 2017;152(1):73–4.

40. Frehywot S, Vovides Y, Talib Z, et al. E-learning in medical education in resource constrained low- and middle-income countries. Hum Resour Health 2013;11:4.

41. ReSurge. Visiting Educator Program. 2018. Available at: https://www.resurge.org/visiting-educators/. Accessed May 21, 2018.

42. Williams B. Cost-benefit analysis. Econ Lab Market Rev 2008;2(12):67.

43. Alkire B, Hughes CD, Nash K, et al. Potential economic benefit of cleft lip and palate repair in Sub-Saharan Africa. World J Surg 2011;35(6): 1194–201.

44. Corlew DS. Estimation of impact of surgical disease through economic modeling of cleft lip and palate care. World J Surg 2010;34(3):391–6.

45. Kotagal M, Agarwal-Harding KJ, Mock C, et al. Health and economic benefits of improved injury prevention and trauma care worldwide. PLoS One 2014;9(3):e91862.

46. Escobar CPM. Cost benefit analysis, value of a statistical life and culture: challenges for regulation. Vniversitas 2007;113. Available at: https://papers.ssrn.com/sol3/papers.cfm?abstract_id=1023496.

47. Higgins AM, Harris AH. Health economic methods: cost-minimization, cost-effectiveness, cost-utility, and cost-benefit evaluations. Crit Care Clin 2012; 28(1):11–24.

48. Alkire B, Vincent J, Meara J. Benefit-cost analysis of a cleft lip and palate surgical subspecialty hospital in India. In: Debas H, Donkor P, Kruk M, et al, editors. Disease control priorities in developing countries. 3rd Edition. Washington, DC: World Bank; 2014.

49. Corlew DS. Economic modeling of surgical disease: a measure of public health interventions. World J Surg 2013;37(7):1478–85.

50. Jakovljevic M, Getzen TE. Growth of global health spending share in low and middle income countries. Front Pharmacol 2016;7:21.

51. Casey KM. The global impact of surgical volunteerism. Surg Clin North Am 2007;87(4):949–60.

52. Billig JI, Lu Y, Momoh AO, et al. A nationwide analysis of cost variation for autologous free flap breast reconstruction. JAMA Surg 2017;152(11): 1039–47.

53. Hamlat CA, Arbabi S, Koepsell TD, et al. National variation in outcomes and costs for splenic injury and the impact of trauma systems: a population-based cohort study. Ann Surg 2012;255(1): 165–70.

54. Kilic A, Shah AS, Conte JV, et al. Understanding variability in hospital-specific costs of coronary artery bypass grafting represents an opportunity for standardizing care and improving resource use. J Thorac Cardiovasc Surg 2014;147(1):109–16.

55. Harris CR, Osterberg EC, Sanford T, et al. National variation in urethroplasty cost and predictors of extreme cost: a cost analysis with policy implications. Urology 2016;94:246–54.

56. Semer NB, Sullivan SR, Meara JG. Plastic surgery and global health: How plastic surgery impacts the global burden of surgical disease. J Plast Reconstr Aesthet Surg 2010;63(8):1244–8.

57. Deckelbaum DL, Gosselin-Tardif A, Ntakiyiruta G, et al. An innovative paradigm for surgical education programs in resource-limited settings. Can J Surg 2014;57(5):298–9.

58. Bryant J. Health and the developing world. Ithaca (NY): Cornell University Press; 1969. London.

59. Contini S, Taqdeer A, Cherian M, et al. Emergency and essential surgical services in Afghanistan: still a missing challenge. World J Surg 2010;34(3):473–9.

60. Farmer PE, Kim JY. Surgery and global health: a view from beyond the OR. World J Surg 2008; 32(4):533–6.

61. Hutton G, Rehfuess E, Organization WH. Guidelines for conducting cost-benefit analysis of household energy and health interventions. Geneva (Switzerland): World Health Organization; 2006.

62. Cookson R, Dolan P. Principles of justice in health care rationing. J Med Ethics 2000;26(5):323–9.

63. Cookson R, Dolan P. Public views on health care rationing: a group discussion study. Health Policy 1999;49(1–2):63–74.

Developing a Sustaining Program of Surgical Care in the Developing World

Kavitha Ranganathan, MD*, Krishnan Raghavendran, MBBS

KEYWORDS

- Global surgery • Sustainability • Research in global surgery • Developing global surgery

KEY POINTS

- The global burden of surgical disease processes continues to grow due to the increase in chronic disease processes and persistent impact of trauma.
- The creation of sustainable surgical care requires the development of clinical infrastructure, educational initiatives, and research.
- Multidisciplinary care amongst surgeons, anesthesiologists, nurses, and other personnel is critical for safe perioperative care.
- Laboratory and blood bank facilities are important adjunctive services to optimize surgical safety.

INTRODUCTION

Previously labeled the "stepchild" of global health, the field of Surgery has remained relatively obscure in terms of its application to health care in low- and middle-income countries.[1,2] Due to the prevalence of infectious diseases including malaria, human immunodeficiency virus (HIV), and tuberculosis, life expectancy in regions plagued by these epidemics was quite low; consequently the need to improve access to surgical care was overshadowed by the devastating impact of these diseases. More recently, however, as a result of successful interventions targeted against these conditions, life expectancy has increased. The role of surgery in the treatment of cardiovascular diseases, gynecologic disorders, trauma, and malignancy to overcome the overwhelming discrepancy between the need for surgery and the current lack of access has now come to light.[3]

The burden of surgical diseases accounts for at least 11% of the overall global burden of disease. More than 5 billion people lack access to safe surgical care, with more than 2 billion of these people lacking access to any form of surgery regardless of safety considerations. Because of this lack of access, more than 17 million people will die each year of surgically treatable conditions; surgically treatable diseases have overtaken infectious conditions as the main cause of death in many regions of the world. There is a current estimated deficit of 143 million procedures each year.[4] In this article, the authors review the needs and processes required to develop sustainable surgical systems in low resource environments.

CLINICAL CONSIDERATIONS FOR SUSTAINABLE SURGICAL SYSTEMS

The first step in developing sustainable surgical systems is to acknowledge the multidisciplinary nature of care that is required in the management of any surgical patient. Proper preoperative, intraoperative, and postoperative care necessitates the participation of anesthesiologists, nurses, primary care physicians, and surgeons.[1] In addition, challenges must be overcome in infrastructure

The authors have nothing to disclose.
Department of Surgery, University of Michigan, 1500 East Medical Center Drive, Ann Arbor, MI 48105, USA
* Corresponding author.
E-mail address: krangana@med.umich.edu

Hand Clin 35 (2019) 391–395
https://doi.org/10.1016/j.hcl.2019.07.002

development, laboratory supplies, physical equipment, supply chain management, and equipment maintenance.[5] Although initially daunting to develop such extensive teams, countries that have prioritized this initial investment have also realized coincident benefits to the rest of the health care system, given the concomitant improvement in care for other patients requiring complex nursing care, blood banks, and laboratory facilities.[5,6] Justman and colleagues[7] note the spillover effects of improving laboratory systems for the care of patients with HIV through the United States President's Emergency Plan for AIDS Relief–related initiatives into other areas of the health system. Once such systems have been built, additional questions surrounding the maintenance of international standards of care, quality, and reliability persist. Strengthening Laboratory Management Toward Accreditation (SLMTA) and the Stepwise Laboratory Improvement Process Towards Accreditation (SLIPTA) are examples of programs that have been implemented in low- and middle-income countries to enhance the quality and reliability of laboratory diagnostic findings. SLMTA is a program that provides mentorship to laboratory managers to continue facility development in low-resource environments; SLIPTA is a program that audits laboratory systems to ensure ongoing quality care.[8] The implementation of these programs has resulted in laboratory infrastructure improvements across many countries in Africa. For example, before the utilization of these programs in 2009, South Africa was the only accredited country in all of Africa with regard to laboratory facilities. In 2017, after the implementation of these programs, 54 laboratories have become accredited in more than 49 countries and more than 5000 people have received training across the continent.[5] Ongoing commitments from local governments and donor organizations in both the public and private sector are necessary to ensure the sustainability of such programs.[9]

The presence of a blood bank is also critical to ensure surgical safety, particularly in centers managing a high volume of trauma.[10] In a systematic review by Raykar and colleagues,[11] limitations including insufficient blood donation due to poor health infrastructure, low awareness of donation practices, and social stigma have limited the ability to develop such systems in low- and middle-income countries. The average donation rate in low-income countries is 2.8 per 1000 people, whereas that in high-income countries is more than 36 per 1000 people.[12] Donation rates in low- and middle-income countries are likely overestimates because they do not account for blood

that is infected by HIV, hepatitis B virus, or parasitic disease processes.[13,14] Because no specific interventions have revolutionized the blood bank industry in low-income countries to date, ongoing ideas and innovations to improve the current state of access to blood are critical.

Establishing proper preoperative and postoperative evaluation protocols is essential to the practice of safe surgery. Although many of the most essential surgical services including trauma, obstetric, and cancer care are delivered in urgent or emergent settings, standardizing preoperative algorithms of care optimizes outcomes despite resource scarcity. Given the relative scarcity of health care providers in most of the world, anesthesiologists commonly serve as primary care providers in the preoperative setting.[15] Unfortunately, little data exist on the number of anesthesia providers in most low-income countries. In fact, nonphysician providers make up the largest proportion of anesthesia providers in many of these regions due to brain drain and inadequate compensation for anesthesiologists.[1] To ensure safety during the administration of general anesthesia, pulse oximeters are a minimum requirement. Task shifting to nonphysician providers may optimize care in the absence of anesthesiologists; nursing staff can be trained to detect common postoperative complications including signs of bleeding and cardiopulmonary instability that may require reintubation or return to the operating room in the immediate postoperative setting. Pharmaceutical companies must continue to evaluate the potential benefits of reducing the price of drugs in low-income countries to benefit the population at large.

To optimize sustainability of surgical care in low-resource environments, we must also consider the potential impact of postsurgical complications. Surgical site infections (SSIs) are the most common complication acquired in the health care setting, accounting for 38% of all nosocomial infections each year.[16] SSIs are a major cause of morbidity and mortality and contribute significantly to the economic burden of postsurgical care and antibiotic resistance patterns both nationally and internationally.[17,18] Although many factors including surgical technique, duration of surgery, and patient comorbidities are known to affect the likelihood of developing a surgical site infection, preoperative antibiotic prophylaxis is one of the most effective, easily documented, and modifiable measures available to decrease the incidence of SSIs. Thus, the proper use, timing, and duration of antibiotic therapy are critically important to consider when expanding access to surgery in a safe and effective manner in resource-limited regions. Instituting standardized practices of preoperative antibiotic prophylaxis procurement and administration are critical components of a safe surgical environment. As patients in low-income countries are 9 times more likely to develop a surgical site infection than those in high-income countries, it is imperative that resources are also allocated for prophylaxis against SSIs to ensure sustainability.[19] These policies are important not only for surgery-specific environments but also for health care systems in general, as the consequences of worsening patterns of antibiotic resistance, costs of readmission and reoperation, and economic burden of care are widespread and far-reaching.[20] In addition, the local bacteriology and existence of multidrug-resistant bacteria add to the complexity of prescribing the correct antibiotic. The most serious consequence of not establishing guidelines and resources for preoperative antibiotic prophylaxis in a preemptive fashion is the development and expansion of antibiotic resistance. Although overall antibiotic use has increased by 36% in low- and middle-income countries, the quality of antibiotics prescribed is often unregulated and the second-line antibiotics required in the setting of drug resistance are either unavailable or unaffordable.[21] Antibiotic stewardship programs and adherence to strict guidelines for prescription of antibiotics are an absolute must. When a patient presents with a postsurgical infection, prompt and correct diagnosis, proper antibiotic agent selection, availability of diagnostic studies and operating rooms, and accessibility of intravenous fluids and other pharmacologic adjuncts are the minimum requirements for recovery. In resource-limited environments, variable access to antibiotics, improper regulation of drug pricing, lack of diagnostic modalities to detect deep space infections, and limited availability of providers able to promptly recognize and treat SSIs invariably manifest as high mortality rates and profound losses in productivity as a result of the morbidity incurred.[22] As a result, the development of postsurgical infections predisposes to the progression of multidrug-resistant organisms not only among surgical patients, but across all patients, providers, and communities in contact with this population.[20]

EDUCATIONAL CONSIDERATIONS FOR SUSTAINABLE SURGICAL SYSTEMS

Any successful, sustainable model of surgical care must also foster the education of its future workforce. Training medical students, residents, nurses, and other personnel is a critical component of this process. Although local training programs are more favorable to implement, this can be difficult given the high initial costs required. Importantly, local training programs limit the potential impact of brain drain or the inclination of local health care workers to emigrate from the home country to more urban, high-resource environments. Although the inclusion of international collaborators or institutions for training in developed countries may offset costs, this can unfortunately entice physicians to stay in the host country. Internal brain drain is another factor to consider; without proper governmental support to public hospital systems, physicians and other members of the health care team may migrate to private practice settings where compensation is greater and quality of life potentially better. Those interested in developing sustainable models of surgical care must be aware of these limitations. If approached thoughtfully, however, such collaborations can provide life-changing opportunities for trainees in both high- and low-resource environments. For example, through a collaboration with the University of Michigan, Ethiopian surgeons are now performing kidney transplants under a specialized, longitudinal training program within Ethiopia.[23] Conversely, for those in high-income countries, trainees who partake in clinical rotations abroad are more likely to continue to contribute to health care systems internationally than those who have not had these experiences.

Mission trips represent a controversial form of surgical care delivery due to the potential impact on surgeons and patients in low- and middle-income countries. If appropriately designed to include capacity building, mission trips can serve as a way to educate local physicians and surgeons in the management of complications, surgical techniques, and perioperative care. Local health care workers must participate from the beginning to define the needs of the community. Including medical students, residents, and nursing staff is also critical to ensure optimal knowledge transmission. Without the inclusion of local members of the community the goal to achieve sustainability cannot be met.

SUSTAINING SURGICAL SYSTEMS THROUGH RESEARCH

To ensure continued development and quality improvement, research is a critical component of sustainability.[24] For international institutions interested in developing surgical care in low- and middle-income countries and for health care systems with new or nonexistent surgical systems, understanding the needs of the community from an epidemiologic perspective, implementing published, proven pathways of improving access to surgical care, and measuring progress over time through research is of utmost importance. For international institutions in high-income countries and for health care systems in low-resource environments, symbiotic collaborations form the foundation of success. Developing relationships is the first step in this process; successful initiatives within other fields particularly in the management of HIV, malaria, and tuberculosis were founded on this principle. It is equally important to understand the local environment and the prevailing culture at the foreign institutions. Building such a collaborative relationship takes time and varies with the host country involved. Such collaborations take many years to develop and must focus on the needs of the local hospital to be successful. At the University of Michigan, the authors recently described the creation of a clinical and research collaborative with the All India Institute of Medical Sciences.[25] Because institutions in low- and middle-income countries have limited resources and are already overburdened by the volume of patients, research in the form of additional labor may not be feasible. Securing funding in high-resource environments to supplement the effort required in low-resource regions can facilitate this process. Although technological innovations such as telemedicine can facilitate the development of longitudinal relationships over time, there must also be a direct, tangible benefit to the community at hand. Thus, ensuring a common goal is of utmost importance.

Once the collaboration is established, it is important to define a focus based on the needs of the target population. For example, in the collaboration between the All India Institute of Medical Sciences (AIIMS) and the University of Michigan, local physicians demonstrated their interest in studying research methods to improve their ability to initiate studies independently. Consequently, a research methods course was crafted by engaging and connecting local physicians at AIIMS with research faculty at the University of Michigan. The course has subsequently fostered the development of grassroots initiatives and research projects that have resulted in grants and papers for participating physicians at AIIMS. It is also important to focus on areas of research pertaining to the local environment. Investigators from the developed world should focus on these problems and help define research questions that are considered meaningful and pertain to the diseases in the low- and middle-income countries. Finally,

the major purpose of these initiatives is to build capacity. For long-term success, funding is critical. Although the National Institutes of Health, Fogarty International Center, and private foundations are potential sources of funding, securing these resources is extremely competitive and oftentimes insufficient to completely meet the local needs. Factors that may distinguish an application include the designation of local community members and/or surgeons as principal investigators in the study design, an established record of publications and/or funding, and applications focused on interventions in addition to defining epidemiologic trends.

SUMMARY

Sustainability in global surgery initiatives requires a stable clinical infrastructure to care for patients, education systems that foster the development of future trainees, and research to support progress and continued evaluation. The development of such systems requires strong collaboration between local health care workers, community members, and international institutions to encourage success in a team-based manner. Ensuring sustainability requires a holistic, targeted approach toward capacity building and promotion of independent clinical care and research.

REFERENCES

1. Meara JG, McClain CD, Rogers SO Jr, et al, editors. Global surgery and anesthesia manual: providing care in resource-limited settings. Florida: CRC Press; 2014.
2. Farmer PE, Kim JY. Surgery and global health: a view from beyond the OR. World J Surg 2008; 32(4):533–6.
3. Meara JG, Greenberg SL. The Lancet Commission on Global Surgery Global surgery 2030: evidence and solutions for achieving health, welfare and economic development. Surgery 2015;157(5):834–5.
4. Weiser TG, Regenbogen SE, Thompson KD, et al. An estimation of the global volume of surgery: a modelling strategy based on available data. Lancet 2008;372(9633):139–44.
5. Nkengasong JN, Yao K, Onyebujoh P. Laboratory medicine in low-income and middle-income countries: progress and challenges. Lancet 2018; 391(10133):1873–5.
6. Horton S, Sullivan R, Flanigan J, et al. Delivering modern, high-quality, affordable pathology and laboratory medicine to low-income and middle-income countries: a call to action. Lancet 2018; 391(10133):1953–64.
7. Justman JE, Koblavi-Deme S, Tanuri A, et al. Developing laboratory systems and infrastructure for HIV

scale-up: A tool for health systems strengthening in resource-limited settings. J Acquir Immune Defic Syndr 2009;52:S30–3.

8. Yao K, McKinney B, Murphy A, et al. Improving quality management systems of laboratories in developing countries: an innovative training approach to accelerate laboratory accreditation. Am J Clin Pathol 2010;134(3):401–9.

9. Shrivastava R, Gadde R, Nkengasong JN. Importance of public-private partnerships: Strengthening laboratory medicine systems and clinical practice in Africa. J Infect Dis 2016;213(suppl_2):S35–40.

10. Raykar NP, Kralievits K, Greenberg SL, et al. The blood drought in context. Lancet Glob Health 2015;3:S4–5.

11. Kralievits KE, Raykar NP, Greenberg SL, et al. The global blood supply: a literature review. Lancet 2015;385:S28.

12. World Health Organization. Global database on blood safety: summary report 2011. Geneva (Switzerland): WHO; 2011.

13. Buyx AM. Blood donation, payment, and non-cash incentives: classical questions drawing renewed interest. Transfus Med Hemother 2009;36(5):329–39.

14. Allain JP. Moving on from voluntary non-remunerated donors: who is the best blood donor? Br J Haematol 2011;154(6):763–9.

15. Holmer H, Lantz A, Kunjumen T, et al. Global distribution of surgeons, anaesthesiologists, and obstetricians. Lancet Glob Health 2015;3:S9–11.

16. April 2013 CDC/NHSN protocol corrections, clarification, and additions. Available at: http://www.cdc.gov/nhsn/PDFs/pscManual/9pscSSIcurrent.pdf. Accessed July 10, 2013.

17. Consensus paper on the surveillance of surgical wound infections. The Society for Hospital Epidemiology of America; The Association for Practitioners in Infection Control; The Centers for Disease Control; The Surgical Infection Society. Infect Control Hosp Epidemiol 1992;13:599.

18. Horan TC, Gaynes RP, Martone WJ, et al. CDC definitions of nosocomial surgical site infections, 1992: a modification of CDC definitions of surgical wound infections. Infect Control Hosp Epidemiol 1992;13:606.

19. WHO Health Care-associated Information Fact Sheet.

20. Laxminarayan R, Duse A, Wattal C, et al. Antibiotic resistance—the need for global solutions. Lancet Infect Dis 2013;13(12):1057–98.

21. Van Boeckel TP, Gandra S, Ashok A, et al. Global antibiotic consumption 2000 to 2010: an analysis of national pharmaceutical sales data. Lancet Infect Dis 2014;14(8):742–50.

22. Becker JU, Theodosis C, Jacob ST, et al. Surviving sepsis in low-income and middle-income countries: new directions for care and research. Lancet Infect Dis 2009;9(9):577–82.

23. Ahmed MM, Tedla FM, Leichtman AB, et al. Organ transplantation in Ethiopia. Transplantation 2019;103(3):449–51.

24. Ranganathan K, Habbouche J, Sandhu G, et al. Cultivating global surgery initiatives abroad and at home. J Grad Med Educ 2018;10(3):258–60.

25. Raghavendran K, Misra MC, Mulholland MW. The role of academic institutions in global health: building partnerships with low-and middle-income countries. JAMA Surg 2017;152(2):123–4.

Overcoming Barriers to Hand Surgical Care in Low-Resource Settings

Andy F. Zhu, MD[a],*, Terry R. Light, MD[b]

KEYWORDS

- Hand surgery • International hand surgery • Low-resource settings
- Low- and middle-income countries • Global outreach • Overcoming barriers

KEY POINTS

- There is a growing need for hand surgical care in low- and middle-income countries.
- Barriers to surgical care exist at the level of the patient, physician, institution, and infrastructure.
- A thorough understanding of a country's needs, resources, and goals are required in planning an outreach initiative.
- It is important to identify the specific model or approach of an outreach initiative.

INTRODUCTION

Over the last several decades, advances in public health have led to a shift in global disease burden from communicable diseases to noncommunicable diseases, particularly in low- and middle-income countries (LMICs).[1,2] With this shift, the *years lived with disability* metric has been used to measure the effect of noncommunicable diseases rather than premature death. In 2010, injury was the second leading cause of disease worldwide and accounted for 11% of all disability-adjusted life years.[3] With continued industrialization and urbanization of LMICs, this percentage is likely to rise and increases the disease burden amenable to surgical intervention.[4] A surge in hand injuries will surely coincide with urbanization as occupational accidents, burns, and road traffic accidents comprise a substantial portion of hand trauma in LMICs.[5,6] Although there is a growing interest in global outreach hand surgery; many challenges and barriers exist.[7,8]

It is estimated that the poorest third of the world's population receive only 3.5% of the 234 million major surgical operations undertaken worldwide.[9] Approximately 95% of the population in LMICs lack access to basic surgical care.[10] Development of a successful and meaningful hand surgery global outreach initiative requires, first and foremost, choosing the approach of the initiative. The approach designates resources, duration, and goals of an initiative, and the most common models include a vertical, horizontal, or diagonal approach. After an approach is chosen, the most common barriers to care must be identified. Because LMICs do not have identical needs, each location must be individually assessed. Barriers can be broadly categorized as patient-related, physician-related, institution-related, and infrastructure-related.[3] Understanding and addressing these barriers is critical to development of an outreach initiative.

MODELS OF OUTREACH SURGERY

It is important at the outset to clearly establish the approach of a hand surgery outreach initiative. This is a complex issue and requires an understanding

Disclosure: Neither author has any conflicts relative to this material.
[a] Department of Orthopaedic Surgery, Loyola University Medical Center, Loyola University Health System, 2160 South First Avenue, Maywood, IL 60153, USA; [b] Department of Orthopaedic Surgery, Loyola Stritch School of Medicine, 2160 South First Avenue, Maywood, IL 60153, USA
* Corresponding author.
E-mail address: tlight@lumc.edu

Hand Clin 35 (2019) 397–402
https://doi.org/10.1016/j.hcl.2019.07.001

of the host country's needs, resources, and availability, as well as the volunteers' focus, resources, and availability. Three well-established approaches or models of outreach initiatives have been defined: vertical, horizontal, and diagonal.[8]

The *vertical approach* provides scalable, efficient surgical care in a timely fashion. These initiatives are typically surgical specialty focused, operate outside of the existing health care system or structure, provide their own resources, and are privately funded.[11] Examples include initiatives in which physicians, nurses, supplies, and operating room facilities are contained on a uniquely equipped aircraft that provides mobile and complete services to a host country. The short project duration of these initiatives is generally attractive to surgical volunteers. The vertical approach is often used in urgent humanitarian response to natural disasters because of its scalability and ability to efficiently deliver surgical supplies and equipment especially in LMICs.[8] A scalable initiative is not limited by host resources and therefore can be quickly expanded as needed, or as funding allows, to meet the needs of a country. Initiatives in response to disasters or epidemics often generate strong donor interest owing to the publicity generated and relatively short-term solutions and outcomes. The vertical approach has also been effectively used, through a combination of vaccinations and education initiatives, by many programs in treating nonsurgical conditions including: HIV/AIDS treatment, polio immunization, tuberculosis control, and male circumcision.[11–13] Disadvantages include its narrow spectrum, uncoordinated interventions, lack of long-term follow-up, and stifling of the development of local hospital structure and building a dependence on outside services.[11,14]

The *horizontal approach* emphasizes long-term investment and development within the health care infrastructure of the country, emphasizing the expansion of publicly funded health care systems.[12,13] Historically the horizontal approach has been implemented to strengthen primary care systems. More recently, infectious disease treatment groups have shifted their focus away from a vertical approach to a horizontal approach.[15] Strengthening of a health care system benefits all patients, builds capacity for long-term change, and may also facilitate disease-specific treatments.[11] Application to surgical treatment requires investment in surgical infrastructure and human capital.[16] Challenges to the development of a health care infrastructure include an extended implementation period, government reliance and cooperation, and difficulty assessing outcomes.

These barriers may dampen interest in private funding.[15] The required long-term commitment limits the appeal of horizontal programs to physicians who have practice and family obligations within their home country.

A diagonal approach is a balanced combination of vertical and horizontal approaches. Ideally, it strengthens the development of a health care infrastructure and provides the immediate services needed by the host country. It focuses not only on providing surgical services but enhancing local trainee experience and cultivating a culture of academic investigation and interdisciplinary care with the end goal of creating a self-sustaining entity.[11] Our craniofacial surgery colleagues continue to successfully implement this approach in the treatment of craniofacial disorders in LMICs.[17] Programs such as Operation Smiles have expanded from solely providing surgical care during its inception in 1982 to development of local business models, educating local professionals, and establishment of medical records.[18]

The diagonal approach is best suited to provide long-term hand surgical care. The additional expertise required to perform safe and effective hand surgery calls on highly trained hand surgeons to provide immediate care to patients while providing a presence to develop and train local surgeons. This continuity of commitment can be achieved by organizations that are able to integrate the skills of rotating health care providers with a consistent institution focus over time.

PATIENT-RELATED BARRIER

Among the many barriers to providing care in LMICs, none are more powerful than patient barriers. Patient health education is often limited in LMICs. Patients may be unaware of treatment options, or even that a condition can be treated surgically. This is often seen in congenital hand conditions for which parents accept their child's condition unaware that reconstructive surgery can provide functional and aesthetic improvement for many children. In addition, a lack of education regarding the value of postsurgical follow-up or rehabilitation can compromise outcomes. Because complex treatments may require a prolonged time away from work, the disruption of income is a barrier to care for many in LMICs.

It is important for a provider to recognize and respect local social and cultural beliefs and not to presume that such beliefs reflect ignorance or lack of education. For example, in some Latin American cultures polydactyly is regarded as a blessing or a symbol of pride. Antonio Alfonseca was a Major League Baseball player with postaxial polydactyly who enjoyed several nicknames including *El Pulpo* (The Octopus). Alternatively, in many Asian cultures retaining the anatomic number of digits is culturally important. In the Cantonese language the word for *four* sounds identical to the word for *death*. Five digits are much preferred to 4 digits because 4 is regarded as an unlucky number. Asian families are thus reluctant to consider deletion of a hypoplastic thumb in favor of a 4-digit hand consisting of 3 fingers and pollicization of the index finger. Discussion of potential benefit of thumb amputation and pollicization will fall on deaf ears. Similar societal beliefs may underlie decisions in some parts of the world to replant a single amputated or crushed digit.[19] An understanding and respect for each patient's needs, culture, and economic situation is necessary for optimal treatment of hand injuries.

Cost, a universal barrier to health care, is particularly important in LMICs. Many studies have demonstrated that financial concerns are the most substantial barrier to accessing subspecialty surgical care.[20] Direct costs related to care include hospital and surgical fees, medications, and transportation. Indirect costs include time off work and the costs of caregivers. Often these expenses are paid directly by the patient and not subsidized or reimbursed by insurance or government.[3] Relatively high costs may deter patients from seeking care even when it could substantially improve their quality of life and function. Although visiting physicians may contribute their time and expertise in care, the costs of additional personnel and supplies to support visitors may be substantial and may require shifting resources from other important health care initiatives. One would not want to divert funds away from basic health care needs, such as childhood inoculations, to support elective hand reconstruction. Such resource judgements must remain the domain of local health care or hospital leadership.

PHYSICIAN-RELATED BARRIERS

The increasing burden of surgical disease in LMICs is accompanied by the growing need for skilled health care professionals. Hand surgery is a specialized field of care. In the United States, well-trained orthopedic, plastic surgery, or general surgical specialists already gain hand surgery expertise by additional training, often a year-long fellowship. In some Scandinavian and Pacific countries, dedicated programs have been established to train hand surgeons without additional years of plastic or orthopedic residency training. Many LMICs not only lack hand surgeons but have a shortage in the surgical workforce in

general. The surgical workforce in many LMICs depends on nonphysicians, including paramedic professionals and nurses.[21,22] Often local surgeons lack formal training in the care of hand injuries and conditions.

Education of local surgeons is an important strategy to improve access to hand surgical care.[8,14] This can be achieved by sending less-experienced surgeons to neighboring cities within the region or to a higher-income country for more advanced surgical education. Aside from the financial cost of advanced physician training, physician emigration to more developed regions or out of LMICs creates a "brain drain" that further strips intellectual power and undermines access to surgical care in LMICs. Short-term traveling fellowships, such as programs sponsored by the American Society for Surgery of the Hand and the American Association for Hand Surgery, provide local surgeons with the opportunity to learn and observe the practice of hand surgery in higher-income countries.

Outreach initiatives can bring highly skilled physicians to local communities to provide surgical care to patients as well as focused education for local physicians. A well-designed program builds a foundation of trust, and learning amplifies local access to specialized surgical care. An initiative must foster a relationship with the local medical community. Visiting surgeons must avoid discord with physicians who may regard the outside physicians as competition, undermining their legitimacy. Although local surgeons may lack specialized training, they should be treated as colleagues and their abilities should not be underestimated. They must be embraced as part of the team and participate in all aspects of patient care because they will be providing follow-up care for shorter-term outreach initiatives. The visiting surgeon should keep open lines of electronic communication after the surgical program has concluded to provide optimal follow-up patient care. This prevents local surgeons and their patients from feeling abandoned. Maintaining open dialogue often leads to future consultation regarding the care of additional patients.

It is, of course, essential that only ethical, informed care is provided. No procedure should be performed if it is not indicated in the visiting surgeon's home country. A lack of resource and limited access to care does not justify inadequate or inferior care. Complex, risky cases may seem the most interesting and challenging but it may be more useful to choose a safer, more straightforward approach that could be replicated by assisting or observing surgeons. A toe-to-thumb transfer may be a technical tour de force, but may not be safely reproduced by less-experienced observing surgeons. Demonstration of surgical procedures are most effective if they illustrate underlying principles of care that can be extended to other procedures.

Learning is a reciprocal process. Outreach experiences are invaluable to the visiting team because they may confront the challenge of treating late-stage or more advanced disease than they encounter in their native countries. Education must also be provided for the local health care team. The education provided should coincide with the resources available to the local surgeon. Techniques involving sophisticated equipment that accompanies the visiting surgeon and leaves with the surgeon, but remains unavailable to local surgeons, may benefit the treated patient but does little to improve the care provided by the local health system.

Volunteering physicians also face obstacles. Outreach initiatives require surgeons to spend time away from their practice while practice overhead expenses continue. Over 80% of surgical trainees report that they are interested in involvement in global surgery.[23] The barriers to participation include funding support, protected time, and institutional recognition of academic contributions.[23] Other barriers include the regulations of the local government in the host country, such as obtaining visas, licenses, and hospital credentials. Personal safety relative to communicable diseases and political stability is essential.

The recent increase in global outreach initiative programs has led to the rapid development of a multibillion-dollar industry, medical *voluntourism*, a phenomenon that has generated much concern.[24] Broadly stated, voluntourism is tourism in which travelers participate in volunteer work. Companies provide packages to often exotic locations selling participants the ability to travel and "volunteering" to help the native population. These companies particularly target young students who are interested in health care because it provides "medical experience" and is a resume builder for applications in an increasingly competitive field. Although there may be some benefit to the host community, the medical ethics behind these programs is of concern. Often untrained and uncertified participants are conducting a greater degree of patient "care" than would be allowed in their home country given their level of experience. Not only can this substandard care be detrimental to the individual patient, but, on an infrastructure level, the growth of entire health systems can be stunted. The presence of "free care" and medications disincentivizes the development of local community health care systems. Reliance on voluntourist programs to deliver consistent health services is not a solution and perpetuates the health care crisis that already disproportionately affects LMICs. It is critical to scrutinize outreach initiatives and to ensure one is "doing good" rather than "feeling good."

INSTITUTION-RELATED BARRIER

Because institution-related barriers are rooted in the economic and political climate, these concerns are inherently complex. Accessibility, staffing, funding, and equipment are a few of the common challenges at the institutional level. These barriers are magnified in LMICs and require long-term investment to produce lasting changes.

The presence of a local hospital with surgical services does not guarantee that a visiting surgeon will gain access to those services. Hospitals in LMICs are often overwhelmed by demand but understaffed and underfunded. This leads to delayed treatment, late referrals, inconsistent follow-up, and suboptimal quality of care.[20] It is not uncommon to see hallways lined with postoperative patients because inpatient rooms are crammed to maximum capacity.

Malunions, nonunions, delayed infections, and large, undiagnosed masses are often encountered in LMICs. When considering a location for a surgical initiative, a thorough discussion with health care providers should consider local hospital capacity. Outreach initiatives should understand that providing staff services, time, and equipment may not be enough. Some hospitals require facility and operating fees to responsibly balance the real cost of "lending" facility resources.

Staffing and funding of care in LMICs are separate but often related issues. Scarcity of funds creates pressure to use under-qualified professionals to provide otherwise unavailable services.[21,22] Interestingly, this is not always an unsuccessful approach as some evidence has shown task shifting in low-income countries can produce similar patient outcomes at lower costs.[16] Education should be directed to all members of the local health care team. Hand therapy, a crucial part of hand care, is often absent in LMICs. Providing nonoperative education is an effective means of improving hand care in a setting with limited surgical resources.

There is a strong demand for functional medical equipment in LMICs. As developed countries continue to adopt new equipment and technologies, old but functional equipment is routinely taken out of service. Some countries rely on nearly 80% of health care equipment to be funded by international donors or foreign governments.[25]

Unfortunately, many generous donations fail to confer the anticipated benefit. It has been estimated that more than half of the equipment donated to LMICs are not used because of lack of spare parts, complexity of equipment maintenance, or lack of proper training in the use of the equipment.[25] In some cases the donated equipment is not appropriate for the specific needs and resources of the recipient country.

Donors need to consider the type of equipment, resources needed to maintain the equipment, and training required to operate the equipment. Sophisticated implant sets may be worthless if fluoroscopy is required for implant insertion but unavailable at the recipient location. Equipment that requires a constant electrical supply of a differing voltage may not be useable or easily modified. Equipment without guides or manuals in the language of the new locale may remain unused.

An attitude that "something is better than nothing" is counterproductive. Shipping of useless materials is a waste. Donors need to consider needs and the opinions of the local medical community. The recipient medical community may be too polite to refuse donated equipment that they will never use. Particular attention needs to be directed toward single-use and date-expired equipment. Ethical dilemmas arise when donating equipment designed for single use to an environment where multiple use is inevitable.[25] Donation of expired drugs, sutures, or single-use equipment suggests a double standard of care and is offensive to the recipient. Equipment deemed unacceptable in the donor country should be viewed similarly in the recipient country.[26] Exceptions may exist, but only with the consent and understanding of local health care providers.

The World Health Organization has outlined 4 underlying principles for good donations.[26] Health care equipment donations should benefit the recipient to the maximum extent possible. Donations should be given with due respect for the wishes and the authority of the recipient, and in conformity with government policies and administrative arrangements of the recipient country. There should be no double standard in quality. If the quality of an item is unacceptable in the donor country, it is also unacceptable as a donation. There should be effective communication between donor and recipient, with all donations made according to a plan formulated by both parties.

INFRASTRUCTURE-RELATED BARRIER

Improving the health care infrastructure and capabilities of the host country is the ultimate goal of visiting health care providers. Hand surgery outreach initiatives should aim to provide access to high quality, sustainable hand surgical care beyond the life cycle of the project. This requires the long-term presence of outreach initiatives coupled with the political commitment and financial investment of the host country. Although the policies of LMICSs are outside the realm of outreach initiatives, visiting health care programs may serve as a valuable resource in the maturation of local health care infrastructure.

The long-term presence of an initiative or organization is key to achieving infrastructure change. Long-term staff or an uninterrupted rotation of health care teams at local hospitals provides continuity of care and ongoing education. Such visits should promote interdisciplinary professional relationships between anesthetists, surgeons, midlevel providers, primary care physicians, and rehabilitation services, while enabling the local workforce to mature. Follow-up visits for surgically treated patients provide additional opportunities for patient education. A consistent emphasis on education and academic culture drives research, higher education, data collection, and outcome analysis at the local level.[11]

Outcomes assessment is desirable to evaluate the quality of care provided and to drive quality improvement initiatives. Development of methods to facilitate outcomes analysis, such as electronic medical records, clinical measurement tools, and a culture of medical documentation, will substantially improve hand surgical care.[11] These infrastructure improvements are applicable to all fields of health care. Improved documentation and communication facilitates efficient collaboration and continuity of care between health care centers, potentially decreasing overall costs to the system. Implementation of electronic medical records by outreach initiatives is not a novel concept, and previous models should be examined and incorporated when applicable.[27]

SUMMARY

There is an increasing global demand for hand surgical care. The unmet need disproportionately affects LMICs because the gap between what is available in high- and low-resource countries continues to grow. As providers of hand care, we possess the ability and skills to improve the lives of many. Diverse outreach initiatives contribute to improving global hand care. If one chooses to contribute through outreach initiatives, it is imperative to thoughtfully consider the barriers to effectively providing care. Responsibly providing hand surgery care and education in LMICs has the potential to improve the lives of the less fortunate and to provide fulfilling experiences for volunteer health care personnel.

REFERENCES

1. Daar AS, Singer PA, Persad DL, et al. Grand challenges in chronic non-communicable diseases. Nature 2007;450(7169):494–6.

2. Murray CJL, Vos T, Lozano R, et al. Disability-adjusted life years (DALYs) for 291 diseases and injuries in 21 regions, 1990-2010: a systematic analysis for the Global Burden of Disease Study 2010. Lancet 2012;380(9859):2197–223.

3. Ologunde R, Maruthappu M, Shanmugarajah K, et al. Surgical care in low and middle-income countries: burden and barriers. Int J Surg 2014;12(8):858–63.

4. Jamison DT, Breman JG, Measham AR, et al, editors. Disease control priorities in developing countries. 2nd edition. Washington (DC): World Bank; 2006.

5. Saw A, Sallehuddin AY, Chuah UC, et al. Comparison of fracture patterns between rural and urban populations in a developing country. Singapore Med J 2010;51(9):702–8.

6. Legbo J, Opara E-K, Yiltok S. Glabrous skin reconstruction of palmar/plantar defects: a case for reconsideration. Niger J Surg Res 2005;7:168–72.

7. Kozin SH. The richness of caring for the poor: the development and implementation of the Touching Hands Project. J Hand Surg Am 2015;40(3):566–75.

8. Chung KY. The role for international outreach in hand surgery. J Hand Surg Am 2017;42(8):652–5.

9. Weiser TG, Regenbogen SE, Thompson KD, et al. An estimation of the global volume of surgery: a modelling strategy based on available data. Lancet 2008;372(9633):139–44.

10. Alkire BC, Shrime MG, Dare AJ, et al. Global economic consequences of selected surgical diseases: a modelling study. Lancet Glob Health 2015;3(Suppl 2):S21–7.

11. Patel PB, Hoyler M, Maine R, et al. An opportunity for diagonal development in global surgery: cleft lip and palate care in resource-limited settings. Plast Surg Int 2012;2012:892437.

12. Barnighausen T, Bloom DE, Humair S. Going horizontal–shifts in funding of global health interventions. N Engl J Med 2011;364(23):2181–3.

13. Msuya J. Horizontal and vertical delivery of health services: what are the trade-offs?. In: World Bank Group, editor. Background papers for the world development report 2004. Washington, DC: World Bank Group; 2003. p. 1–28.

14. Corlew S, Fan VY. A model for building capacity in international plastic surgery: ReSurge International. Ann Plast Surg 2011;67(6):568–70.

15. Barnighausen T, Bloom DE, Humair S. Health systems and HIV treatment in sub-Saharan Africa: matching intervention and programme evaluation strategies. Sex Transm Infect 2012;88(2):e2.

16. Fulton BD, Scheffler RM, Sparkes SP, et al. Health workforce skill mix and task shifting in low income countries: a review of recent evidence. Hum Resour Health 2011;9:1.

17. Zbar RI, Rai SM, Dingman DL. Establishing cleft malformation surgery in developing nations: a model for the new millennium. Plast Reconstr Surg 2000; 106(4):886–9 [discussion: 890–1].

18. Magee WP. Evolution of a sustainable surgical delivery model. J Craniofac Surg 2010;21(5):1321–6.

19. Maroukis BL, Shauver MJ, Nishizuka T, et al. Cross-cultural variation in preference for replantation or revision amputation: societal and surgeon views. Injury 2016;47(4):818–23.

20. Grimes CE, Bowman KG, Dodgion CM, et al. Systematic review of barriers to surgical care in low-income and middle-income countries. World J Surg 2011;35(5):941–50.

21. Taira BR, Cherian MN, Yakandawala H, et al. Survey of emergency and surgical capacity in the conflict-affected regions of Sri Lanka. World J Surg 2010; 34(3):428–32.

22. Iddriss A, Shivute N, Bickler S, et al. Emergency, anaesthetic and essential surgical capacity in the Gambia. Bull World Health Organ 2011;89(8):565–72.

23. Cheung M, Healy JM, Hall MR, et al. Assessing interest and barriers for resident and faculty involvement in global surgery. J Surg Educ 2018;75(1):49–57.

24. Hartman E. Fair trade learning: ethical standards for community-engaged international volunteer tourism. Tourism and Hospitality Research 2014;14(1–2):108–16.

25. Gatrad AR, Gatrad S, Gatrad A. Equipment donation to developing countries. Anaesthesia 2007;62(Suppl 1):90–5.

26. World Health Organization. Guidelines for health care equipment donations. Geneva (Switzerland): World Health Organization; 2000.

27. McQueen KAK, Burkle FM, Al-Gobory ET, et al. Maintaining baseline, corrective surgical care during asymmetrical warfare: a case study of a humanitarian mission in the safe zone of a neighboring country. Prehosp Disaster Med 2007;22(1):3–7 [discussion: 8].

Postoperative Management of Hand Surgery in the Low- and Middle-Income Countries

Jeanne Riggs, BS, OTRL, CHT[a,b], Kevin C. Chung, MD, MS[c,*]

KEYWORDS

- Global surgery • Low- and middle-income countries • Postoperative therapy • Outreach trips
- Hand therapy • Rehabilitation

KEY POINTS

- There is a shortage of therapists in low- to middle-income countries who are trained to manage hand injuries.
- Surgical outreach trips provide the primary source of hand therapy for patients after hand surgery in low- to middle-income countries.
- Direct patient care and the provision of educating local therapists are the aim and responsibility of a therapist as a member of a surgical outreach team.

The challenges of managing postoperative care for patients in resource-limited settings are substantial. The most common challenge for postoperative management of surgical hand care in low- and middle-income countries (LMICs) is the lack of an established occupational and hand therapy specialty. For example, Kenya has an 18-member hand therapy association listed in the International Federation of Societies for Hand Therapy and was established in 2009.[1] In contrast, the American Society of Hand Therapy has garnered 3473 members since its establishment in 1977.[1] Additionally, the lack of robust training for occupational therapists in many LMICs is a major barrier contributing to the lack of hand therapists worldwide.[2] Occupational therapy (OT) is a health profession that is client centered and

focuses on promoting health and well-being through occupation, with a primary goal of enabling people to participate in the activities of everyday life. Hand therapy is a type of rehabilitation performed by an occupational or physical therapist with patients who suffer from conditions affecting the hands and upper extremities and aims to hasten their return to a productive lifestyle. According to the World Health Organization, there is a paucity of skilled rehabilitation practitioners in LMICs, with estimates of fewer than 10 skilled rehabilitation practitioners per 1 million population.[3]

The Hand Therapy Certification Commission is made up of certified hand therapists (CHTs) from a total of 23 countries with only 5 of the countries considered LMICs. Of the 6761 CHTs worldwide, only 29 therapists are in outlying US territories,

Disclosure Statement: The work was supported by a Midcareer Investigator Award in Patient-Oriented Research (2 K24-AR053120-06) to K.C. Chung. The content is solely the responsibility of the authors and does not necessarily represent the official views of the National Institutes of Health.

[a] Michigan Medicine Plastic Surgery Clinic, Domino's Farms, Lobby A, rm 1108, 24 Frank Lloyd Wright Drive, Ann Arbor, MI 48105, USA; [b] Department of Physical Medicine and Rehabilitation, Michigan Medicine, 325 East Eisenhower Parkway, Ann Arbor, MI 48108, USA; [c] Section of Plastic Surgery, University of Michigan Medical School, The University of Michigan Health System, 1500 East Medical Center Drive, 2130 Taubman Center, SPC 5340, Ann Arbor, MI 48109-5340, USA
* Corresponding author.
E-mail address: kecchung@med.umich.edu

Hand Clin 35 (2019) 403–410
https://doi.org/10.1016/j.hcl.2019.07.005

military bases, and other countries. Thus, the vast majority of CHTs reside within the United States.[4] Furthermore, the European Federation of Societies for Hand Therapy represents 1800 therapists. Among the CHTs, 85% originate from an OT background and 14% from a physical therapy background. Physical therapists in contrast to OTs are movement experts who optimize quality of life through prescribed exercise, hands-on care, and patient education. Additionally, only 1% have a degree in both OT and physical therapy.[5] OT is an important component to recovery and returning to independence, especially in an LMIC, when an individual's ability to work may have extreme consequences for themselves and their dependent family members.

Traditionally, global hand surgery trips include a CHT as part of the team, permitting both direct patient care and provision of training for local nonspecialized therapists. The Touching Hands Project is an American Society for Surgery of the Hand program and is funded by the American Foundation for Surgery of the Hand.[6] It is one of several sources of funding to support hand therapists on these surgical trips. The Evelyn Mackin Grant for Education by a Traveling Hand Therapist is another source of funding via the American Hand Therapy Foundation. This grant was created to foster professional relationships throughout the international hand therapy community and increase the visibility and quality of hand and upper limb rehabilitation through education and communication.[7] Furthermore, the Miguel Vargas International Hand Therapy Teaching Award serves as another source of funding to promote an exchange of ideas between an American Association for Hand Surgery hand therapist member and the host country. The educational focus of this grant is meant to provide informative hands-on training to improve patient care and host site education.

The primary mode of hand therapy provided in LMICs is through global hand surgery trips. In addition to a therapist providing direct patient care during the trip for both surgical and nonsurgical patients, trips can be organized so that the training of local staff is a major component for the traveling hand therapist. The Guatemala Healing Hands Foundation fosters the exchange of educational ideas between therapists in the United States and therapists in Guatemala.[8] Despite the various programs to increase the availability and access to hand therapy in LMICs, individuals in these limited-resource settings still experience tremendous challenges. Thus, innovative strategies are imperative for the development of hand therapy programs in resource-limited parts of the world.

MAIN CHALLENGES TO HAND THERAPY CARE

The limited resources in LMICs are an obvious challenge in the management of postoperative care for patients after their hand surgery. Individuals seeking care during surgical outreach trips do not always have the resources to receive proper care. For example, a pediatric patient in Bolivia may miss their surgery as his or her parents deal with the more urgent problem of getting evicted from their home. Furthermore, transportation strikes are not uncommon in LMICs and can be the only mode of transportation for many who do not own a car, so just getting to a therapist for care remains difficult. Infrastructure such as road conditions are often poor and, during the rainy seasons, nearly impossible to navigate.[9] Additionally, individuals in more rural areas have less access to health care resources. The majority of medical professionals in LMICs work in large cities, making accessibility to care difficult for those in rural villages. In Tanzania, for example, 80% of the population lives in rural areas.[10] Thus, a patient who receives surgical care in a main city will endure challenges going back to the urban center to receive postoperative hand therapy. A study of strategies to improve patient follow-up after surgery in sub-Saharan Africa and South Asia suggests that funding and support from a coordinator would ensure good practices for follow-up are encouraged, including cell phone reminders, patient tracking, and travel reimbursement.[11] Positive outcomes with the use of text messages for both reminders and health care service promotions are reported in sub-Saharan Africa.[12] **Fig. 1** shows the various challenges to hand therapy care in LMICs.

Public funding for hand therapy care in LMICs is lacking. For example, some government support exists for patients to receive hand therapy in Honduras; however, this support is only available to patients referred by particular physicians. Otherwise, patients pay for individual services provided to them in LMICs. For example, Teleton is a publicly funded program in which therapists are contracted to provide hand therapy services for patients on a fee-for-service basis. The organization will often waive the fee if the patient is extremely poor. In LMICs, many conditions of the upper extremity require comprehensive hand therapy to ensure optimal outcomes. In Nepal, upper extremity conditions comprise 42% of all injuries, with the most common mechanisms of injury from falls, road traffic injuries, and burns.[13] However, because of the minimal resources for medical and postoperative care, patients often go untreated or undertreated.[14]

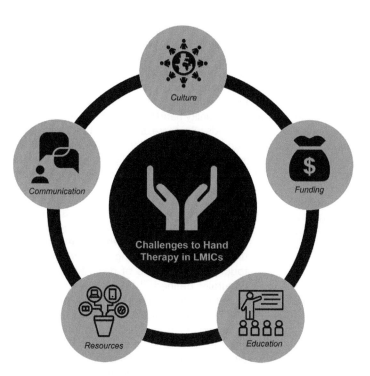

Fig. 1. The various challenges to hand therapy care in LMICs.

Cultural attitudes toward responsibility to achieve a good surgical outcome is a significant challenge in the postoperative treatment for patients receiving surgical treatment in an LMIC.[9] For example, hygiene standards may differ in LMICs, increasing an individual's likelihood of infection. In a systematic review of fracture treatment in LMICs, surgical site infections were found to be more frequent after open reduction and internal fixation in the subgroup of open fractures.[15] Patients need to be taught to take responsibility for their outcome by participating fully in their treatment and exercises at home, including following proper hygiene and wound care. Additionally, a patient may have a poor social support system. This may contribute to further challenges with dressing changes, childcare, or transportation. One patient-related variable that was found to be a barrier to accessing surgical care in Pakistan included a lack of social support.[16] A thorough understanding of the various cultural differences that may contribute to the lack of commitment to achieving a good surgical outcome for postoperative hand therapy will aid in the development of robust therapy systems in LMICs.

Effective patient education is an important component of postoperative hand therapy care. Thus, finding ways to effectively communicate with patients with both a language and cultural barrier may pose an immense challenge. Postoperative instructions may not be followed owing to an incomplete or altered translation provided by an interpreter during outreach efforts. Additionally, an interpreter may not be fluent in a patient's dialect. A patient may speak some English and give a heightened impression of understanding, so strategies should be used to communicate more effectively. These include using shorter sentences with basic words said in a slower, calm voice. Having a pleasant demeanor and a caring smile will help to relax the listener, lowering their anxiety level and making it easier for them to concentrate on the words being spoken.[9] Additionally, there are various technologies to help facilitate the translation in a foreign setting that can be used such as translation apps on a smart phone that offer both audio and written translations.

Communication remains among the most challenging barriers to postoperative hand therapy. Postoperative hand therapy commonly occurs 1 day after the surgery is performed on surgical outreach trips. A patient's bulky postoperative dressing is removed and a smaller compressive dressing applied with family members present. Often an interpreter is not available, so a visiting hand therapist may need to use a translation booklet such as the English/Spanish Phrase Book for Hand Therapists,[17] or a translation app on their phone. A protective orthosis may be fabricated and a home exercise program initiated, using handouts provided by the therapist, which should be in the native language and emphasize pictures and diagrams. A patient may be illiterate and unable to understand written instructions, thus making diagram-emphasized handouts important. Plans are discussed with each patient as far as follow-up with the local surgeon and possible therapy visits; however, this is often not feasible owing to poor resources. For example, a physician involved in surgical outreach trips found that only 25% of patients with machete injuries returned for follow-up care.[18] Identifying ways to improve the number of patients seeking follow-up care will help to improve outcomes for patients in LMICs. Communication is sometimes impossible once a patient returns home and the visiting organization leaves the host country, making it difficult for the patient to receive all the postoperative care needed. Thus, an influential family member may decide that the patient should substitute Western approaches to illness with local customs or follow a particular spiritual belief system.[10]

PROVIDING COST-EFFECTIVE HAND THERAPY CARE

Obstacles permit the opportunity for creativity and innovation for effective hand therapy care that helps to maximize functional outcomes. An important element of innovation for low-resource settings is the ability to meet a specific need. In addition, a device should be affordable and easily

replaceable.[19] In this next section, a short-term surgical outreach trip will be the model discussed when managing the postoperative care. **Fig. 2** illustrates the various ways to provide cost-effective hand therapy care in LMICs.

Patient education is a vital component in providing quality hand therapy. When an individual understands why there are surgical precautions or why hand therapists ask them to wear a protective orthosis, compliance typically will improve. Here are some strategies to use when providing patient education in an LMIC:

- An important aspect of caring for an individual in another part of the world is having cultural competence, which means to understand the meaning of hand gestures, touch, and activities of daily living that are culturally defined.[20] There are many websites that will provide information on the culture, customs, and etiquette of a country including meeting/greeting etiquette, gift giving etiquette, customary punctuality, use of eye contact, and standards of personal space, dress, gestures, taboos, and gender issues.[21,22]
- Patient educational handouts should primarily consist of pictures and diagrams. Additionally, there should be only minimal use of the native

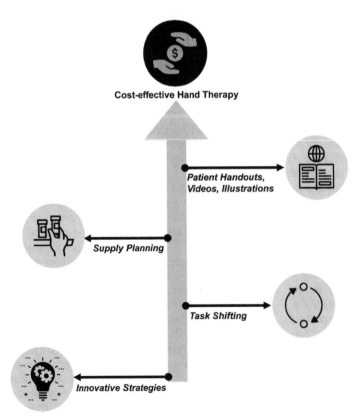

Fig. 2. Cost-effective techniques for providing hand therapy in LMICs.

language. Handouts can be modified with the help of a hospital translator or the therapists can use available materials on various subjects, such as shoulder exercises or hand strengthening exercises, in the appropriate language. Handouts are commonly created for outreach efforts and may be available to a therapist through the outreach organization.

- Pictures and videos are worth a thousand words. Taking an intraoperative video to show the patient after a surgical procedure, such as a tenolysis or contracture release, may demonstrate the improved arc of motion achieved in surgery. This can encourage an individual to reach his or her full potential during postoperative therapy. This is similar to wide awake surgery when a patient can actively move the fingers intraoperatively and witness the improved range of motion gained from the procedure.

Task shifting is the rational redistribution of tasks among health workforce teams and originated in income-poor countries. For example, task shifting includes transferring defined health care tasks, such as dressing changes, traditionally performed by a nurse, to less skilled, but appropriately trained individuals, such as a technician or even a family member.[20] This process can be accomplished by involving the family in postoperative care and may include teaching them surgery precautions, techniques in wound care, donning and doffing orthoses, range of motion exercises, and functional activities as part of a home exercise program. Task shifting has been found to be successful in LMICs in the areas of nurse anesthetists and nonphysician clinicians.[19]

Strategies for best practice in a resource-limited environment are sometimes created out of necessity. A group of senior mechanical engineering students at the University of Michigan are working on creating a low-cost, low-weight hand and wrist rehabilitation device for patients at a hospital in Kumasi, Ghana. It will be used for at-home rehabilitation after hand and wrist injuries and they are consulting with a local physiotherapist.[23] This collaboration came about as a way to improve patient outcomes in an environment where patients are unable to attend therapy as recommended and will permit independent self-stretching and strengthening in a graded manner. A local physiotherapist in Bolivia demonstrated the use of a carpal tunnel splint, which consisted of a 1-inch strip of orthoplast fit from the palm to the distal forearm and applied with 2 straps. This approach is much simpler than in the United States, but limited orthosis material necessitated

its simplicity. Here are some concepts to consider while working in an LMIC that have been recommended and used during surgical outreach trips:

- For pediatric patients, when fitting orthoses, consider if they will need it for the next 6 months or year and fit it accordingly with room for growth on the sides and distally. Extra Velcro straps should be provided for use when expected wear and tear of the original straps occurs.
- Postoperative orthoses may be fabricated before surgery to ease the patient's trauma of trying to do so when they are in pain and likely scared. This strategy is especially effective for a pediatric patient.
- A pediatric patient can be put in a cast while still under anesthesia, then the cast bivalved with a cast saw, and self-adhesive tape applied to keep it intact. This strategy can make their first postoperative visit less scary by avoiding the use of the cast saw while awake.
- A patient may need to use their teeth for removing an orthosis out of necessity. Thus, keeping the straps longer, in this case, will increase their ease of independence. Another orthosis strapping adaptation is to keep the straps longer and to cut a hole at the end so that an individual with bilateral thumb arthritis, for example, can avoid forceful pinch to don and doff their orthosis, but rather slip a finger in the loop to remove.
- Patients should be educated in performing contrast baths for edema control and pain management because some may not have access to microwaves, heating pads, or ice. Typically, this process consists of alternating between warm and cold water soaks for approximately 15 minutes.

Limited space for supplies on surgical outreach trips can lead to creative practices. Although some trips permit for early shipping of supplies directly to the host facility, others limit each team member to 2 pieces of luggage, including personal belongings and supplies to be used on the trip. In a recent article, the creation of a central database was suggested to improve communication between trip organizers, permitting the sharing of information about upcoming trips, site logistics, and personnel or supply needs.[24] In addition to materials used for orthosis fabrication, wound care, and edema control, assistive devices are another supply that is in need in LMICs. The World Health Organization estimates that only 5% to 15% of people with disabilities have access to assistive devices.[15]

The Global Co-operative on Assistive Health Technology aims to improve access to affordable devices globally.[25] Consider using the following suggestions for cost-effective hand therapy on a surgical outreach trip. When supplies are the limiting factor, use local, household items:

- Use inexpensive materials that may be found locally such as putting rice in a sock to create a hot pack for use in a microwave. This strategy can help to facilitate range of motion and pain reduction. Rice is also an effective contact particle in desensitization exercises.
- Health care providers in Kumasi, Ghana, suggest having the patient work on grip and pinch strength using household items such as stacking cups tightly, unscrewing a jar, turning a key in a lock, using clothespins, and buttoning clothing.
- Slings can be made out of discounted remnants from a fabric store or inexpensive sheets for postoperative use.[26]
- An inexpensive in-hand manipulation activity can be made by cutting up a sponge into small cubes.

Cut costs by bringing less expensive items to use rather than items found in a medical catalog:

- Clothespins, silly putty or Play-Doh, which is less expensive than Theraputty, can be used for grip and pinch strengthening.
- A tennis ball may be effectively used between a wall and the painful neck or back for trigger point therapy for factory workers with pain from postural demands and repetitive activities.
- Office rubber bands may be used for strengthening hand intrinsic muscles.

Bring items that have a high likelihood of being reused by local therapy staff:

- Single-use materials are frequently resterilized for repeated use; leave behind your suture removal kits for future use.[27]
- Baoding balls are the traditional metal Chinese balls that are intended to improve finger dexterity and in-hand manipulation. Golf balls may be used in a similar manner.
- Laminated patient educational materials that emphasize diagrams and are in the native language can provide a resource for the local therapist.

While participating in a surgical outreach trip, an individual can help to impact the community and enhance their own experience in the host country. With additional planning and preparation, one may have the opportunity to improve the quality of life for a factory worker or bring a smile to an orphan's face. Textile factories make Honduras Central America's top textile exporter. Workers become experts in the use of sewing machines to create cotton t-shirts and fleece wear. As a therapist, it can be eye opening to observe thousands of workers in a large space, working in small groups to create the various components of a garment. There is no way to reduce the same repetitive movements for a worker; it is much more efficient and cost-effective to have an individual stay in 1 role. Visiting a local industry to evaluate current practices and meet with medical staff can be beneficial in influencing change to reduce or prevent work-related injuries. Furthermore, improving work-related public awareness and incorporating behavioral and environmental modifications make up the primary prevention for hand injuries.[28]

Another opportunity for a visiting therapist to impact the community is to visit orphanages to better understand the community and develop trust between themselves and the local medical staff and patients. This visit may be prearranged and gifts of useful household and personal items, as well as games, are much appreciated. Additionally, by immersing yourself in the local customs, you may gain the trust and respect of your patients and the local medical staff. This may include sharing local cuisine or a beverage with staff, or visiting a local landmark, church, or listening to local music while providing therapy. Learning key therapy words and appropriate greetings in the native language are important elements as well when interacting with patients and staff.

HOW TO IMPROVE LOCAL THERAPIST KNOWLEDGE BASE AND TRAINING

In addition to providing direct patient care, most hand therapists on hand surgery outreach trips participate in teaching. Providing formal lectures and training for local staff is an effective way to improve the knowledge base and skills of these therapists and improve the quality of patient care. The Guatemala Healing Hands Foundation provides educational clinic sessions, and ReSurge International provides formal lectures, which are shared with local therapists. Additional organizations promoting the training of local staff are the Hand Rehabilitation Foundation[7] and Hand Help, Inc. Reaching out to local therapists and schools can maximize training opportunities.

Topics such as orthosis fabrication, therapy protocols, anatomy, diagnoses, therapy, treatment, and surgical techniques may be discussed and demonstrated through less formal means such as observation and one-on-one instruction. Cotreating a patient during clinic is another opportunity to demonstrate new techniques and observe a therapist's skill set and learn from his or her management of the patient. By listening to a local therapist's ideas and techniques, one can provide alternate management ideas in a sharing environment. Local therapists must be empowered to care for patients once the surgical team departs. The sharing of ideas, rather than dictating a treatment plan, can nurture a provider–patient relationship and help them to be independent. However, there may be resource limitations in the application of new knowledge and skills, including a lack of equipment and/or supplies.[29]

Educating staff on injury prevention is another important topic to consider. In terms of hand burns in LMICs, prevention is the most cost-effective strategy. But early treatment when a burn does occur is another public education point because early intervention can have an important impact on decreasing the severity of many hand burns.[30] Additionally, local hand therapists may benefit from attending national hand therapy educational meetings. Thus, sponsoring therapists in an LMIC could permit them to provide more diverse care to patients in their country. Furthermore, donating educational publications in their native language could help to provide educational resources for those without the ability to travel to such meetings. Finally, communication with future outreach therapists as to the needs of the local therapy staff is imperative in helping provide hand therapists with the proper resources. This goal can be accomplished by completing a thorough trip report and/or by making yourself available to communicate before subsequent trips.

SUMMARY

A therapist on a hand surgery outreach trip may contribute by enhancing the lives of patients, impacting the community in a positive way, and creating lifelong memories. Moreover, a therapist can add to the knowledge and skills of local therapists. With improvements in record keeping during surgical outreach trips, therapists can begin to make contributions in regards to measuring and documenting patient outcomes. The majority of current research neglects injury prevention and tends to focus on life-threatening conditions, rather than the impact and lifelong potential disability related to hand injuries.[27] Attention to and funding for research, prevention, and treatment of hand injuries in LMICs need to be a priority to develop strategies in reducing the economic impact of disability in LMICs.[27]

ACKNOWLEDGMENTS

The authors thank Jacob S. Nasser for his help with article editing, organization, and illustrations.

REFERENCES

1. International Federation of Societies of Hand Therapy Membership. Available at: https://www.ifsht.org/country. Accessed April 15, 2019.
2. Deva P. Psychiatric rehabilitation and its present role in developing countries. World Psychiatry 2006;5:164–5.
3. World Health Organization. Rehabilitation 2030: a call for action. Available at: http://www.who.int/disabilities/care/rehab-2030/en/. Accessed April 24, 2018.
4. Hand Therapy Certification Commission. Who is a certified hand therapist?. Available at: https://www.htcc.org/consumer-information/the-cht-credential/who-is-a-cht. Accessed April 15, 2019.
5. European Federation of Societies for Hand Therapy certification. Available at: https://www.eurohandtherapy.org/efsht/echt/. Accessed April 15, 2019.
6. American Society of Surgery for the Hand. Available at: http://www.assh.org/touching-hands. Accessed March 24, 2019.
7. American Hand Therapy Foundation Evelyn Mackin grant. Available at: https://www.ahtf.org/grants/evelyn-mackin-grant/. Accessed April 15, 2019.
8. Guatemala Healing Hands Foundation. Available at: https://www.guatemalahands.org/about. Accessed April 15, 2019.
9. Kolkin J. A physician's perspective on volunteering overseas… It's not all about sharing the latest technology. J Hand Ther 2014;27:152–7.
10. Curci M. Surgical care in developing countries- the limitations of volunteerism, poster presentation, 92nd annual New England Surgical Society. Available at: http://meeting.nesurgical.org/abstracts/2011/P11.cgi. Accessed April 15, 2019.
11. Kishiki E, van Dijk K, Courtright P. Strategies to improve follow-up of children after surgery for cataract: findings from child eye health tertiary facilities in sub-Saharan Africa and South Asia. Eye 2016;30:1234–41.
12. Bright T, Felix L, Kuper H, et al. A systematic review of strategies to increase access to health services among children in low and middle income countries. BMC Health Serv Res 2017;17:252.
13. Gupta S, Wong EG, Nepal S, et al. Injury prevalence and causality in developing nations: results from a countrywide population-based survey in Nepal. Surgery 2015;157:843–9.

14. Bright T, Wallace S, Kuper H. A systematic review of access to rehabilitation for people with disabilities in low- and middle-income countries. Int J Environ Res Public Health 2018;15 [pii:E2165].

15. McQuillan TJ, Cai LZ, Corcoran-Schwartz I, et al. Surgical site infections after open reduction internal fixation for trauma in low and middle human development index countries: a systematic review. Surg Infect (Larchmt) 2018;19:254–63.

16. American Society of Hand Therapists. Store: books. Available at: https://www.asht.org/store. Accessed April 15, 2019.

17. Irfan FB, Irfan BB, Spiegel DA. Barriers to accessing surgical care in Pakistan: healthcare barrier model and quantitative systematic review. J Surg Res 2012;176:84–94.

18. Johnson AR. Machete injuries in Honduras 2019 Philadelphia Hand Symposium presentation. Available at: http://www.handfoundationconference.org/index.php/article-2. Accessed on April 15, 2019.

19. Oppong FC. Innovation in income-poor environments. Br J Surg 2015;102:102–7.

20. Black RM. Cultural considerations of hand use. J Hand Ther 2011;24:104–11.

21. Cultural crossing guide. Available at: guide.culturecrossing.net. Accessed on April 15, 2019.

22. Commisceo Global country guides. Available at: https://www.commisceo-global.com/resources/country-guides. Accessed April 15, 2019.

23. D'Souza K, Linn S, Mosier J, et al. At-home rehabilitation device for hand and wrist injuries in low-resource settings. Mechanical engineering 450, Fall 2018 semester final report.

24. Medoff S, Freed J. The need for formal surgical global health programs and improved mission trip coordination. Ann Glob Health 2016;82:634–8.

25. World Health Organization assistive devices/technologies. What WHO is doing. Available at: http://www.who.int/disabilities/technology/activities/en/. Accessed July 18, 2018.

26. Harvard health publishing. Emergencies and first aid. Available at: https://www.health.harvard.edu/pain/emergencies-and-first-aid-how-to-make-a-sling. Accessed March 24, 2019.

27. Raykar NP, Yorlets RR, Liu C, et al. The how project: understanding contextual challenges to global surgical care provision in low-resource settings. BMJ Glob Health 2016;1:e000075.

28. Siotos C, Ibrahim Z, Bai J, et al. Hand injuries in low- and middle-income countries: systematic review of existing literature and call for greater attention. Public Health 2018;162:135–46.

29. Bodnar BE, Claassen CW, Solomon J, et al. The effect of a bidirectional exchange on faculty and institutional development in a global health collaboration. PLoS One 2015;10:e0119798.

30. Brown M, Chung KC. Post burn contractures of the hand. Hand Clin 2017;33:317–31.

Teaching Hand Surgery in the Developing World
Utilizing Educational Resources in Global Health

Peter Deptula, MD[a],*, Kathleen Chang[b,1], James Chang, MD[a,1]

KEYWORDS

- Surgical education • Global surgery • Surgical capacity • Teaching hand surgery
- Developing world

KEY POINTS

- Teaching hand surgery in the developing world can improve global surgical capacity.
- Hand surgery problems in the developing world are different from those in high-income countries (HICs).
- Principles of an effective curriculum include employing the best teachers, modeling HIC operating room safety, teaching equivalent level of care, sustainability, and the identification and certification of trainees.
- Components of a model curriculum include expert surgeon faculty, a competency-based curriculum, a milestone assessment tool, hands-on training, digital training, and certification.

The greatest burden of global surgical disease is shouldered by low-income and middle-income countries (LMICs).[1,2] Unfortunately, these countries often are ill equipped to manage this burden in its entirety. In response, the global community is resetting its focus on the development of surgical capacity worldwide. This task includes the development of surgeons, anesthesiologists, nurses, surgical technologists, and therapists as well as maintaining supplies and functional facilities.[2,3]

One aspect of building surgical capacity in LMICs is the fostering of trained local surgeons. Challenges to this task include the lack of local expert faculty, absence of a defined curriculum, no competency-based evaluation systems, few subspecialty training opportunities, and lack of financial support.[4] Despite these challenges, investment in the training of local surgeons in LMICs is critical. The task at hand is developing an effective teaching strategy that will give experts the ability to teach hand surgery in the developing world. This article reviews the state of hand surgery in the developing world and outlines a strategy for an effective hand surgery education program.

HAND SURGERY PROBLEMS IN THE DEVELOPING WORLD

A hand surgeon practicing in the developing world faces a wide range of pathology, which greatly differs from that seen in high-income countries (HICs). Congenital upper extremity problems represent one aspect of a global hand surgeon's practice.[5,6] Data surrounding the incidence of

Disclosure Statement: No disclosures.
[a] Department of Surgery, Division of Plastic and Reconstructive Surgery, Stanford University Medical Center, Stanford, CA 94304, USA; [b] Stanford University, Stanford, CA 94304, USA
[1] Present address: 770 Welch Road, Suite 400, Palo Alto, CA 94304.
* Corresponding author. 770 Welch Road, Suite 400, Palo Alto, CA 94304.
E-mail address: pdeptula@stanford.edu

0749-0712/19/© 2019 Elsevier Inc. All rights reserved.

congenital hand conditions are limited.[7,8] The estimate of the overall incidence of congenital upper extremity anomalies, however, is between 3.4 and 5.3 per 10,000 live births.[8] These conditions include radial longitudinal deficiency, thumb hypoplasia, ulnar longitudinal deficiency, cleft hand, syndactyly, polydactyly, and constriction band syndrome.[5,8] Anomalies must be promptly recognized along with their associated medical syndromes, which result in a 14% to 16% 1-year mortality rate of live-born infants.[8] These congenital hand problems often go untreated as a result of lacking hand surgery capacity in LMICs.[6]

Trauma represents another area that an effective hand surgeon must master in LMICs. Data on the types of hand injuries, causes, costs, and outcomes also are limited in the LMIC setting.[9] In developed countries, hand and wrist injuries comprise approximately 28% to 29% of encounters in the emergency department.[9] In the United States, this percentage translates to 18 million phalangeal injuries, resulting in emergency department and physician visits.[10] It is likely that an even greater number of injuries exists in LMICs.[6] As economic development increases in LMICs, hand injuries are projected to rise.[9]

Rapid industrialization, a common phenomenon in LMICs, plays a role in the high incidence of hand trauma.[11] In Ethiopia, most hand injuries occur at work (75%), frequently the product of human-machine interaction. Most of these injuries are treated nonoperatively, resulting in poor patient satisfaction ratings.[11] A similar trend is seen in Nigeria, where hand injuries were most commonly the result of traffic and machine operation injuries.[12] In Malaysia, 24.9% of industrial injuries involved the wrists and hand, where 47.7% of these were classified as severe injuries.[9,13] A less established system of prevention of occupational injuries may explain this high incidence of hand trauma. For example, Sabitu and colleagues[14] demonstrated that in a population of Nigerian welders, 85.3% sustained work-related injuries, 38% involving the hand. Only 17% of these workers reported the use of protective gloves.[9,14] Lack of a workers' compensation system, prohibitive cost of care, and lack of health insurance systems in LMICs further complicate treatment and outcomes from these traumatic injuries.[9]

One study from an urban referral hospital in Kenya demonstrated a similar trend. Here, hand injuries were largely the result of work or machine-related injury, followed by assault.[15] The investigators noted that the majority of hand trauma involved open injuries. The majority of fractures involved the phalanges, followed by the metacarpals and carpal bones. Tendon and nerve injuries were found in 17% and 2% of patients, respectively. In cases of tendon injuries, flexor tendons were affected more often than extensor tendons. Other sources suggest that tendon-related trauma is as high as 50% in those cases presenting to hand clinics in LMICs.[16]

The phenomena of machete-related injury is not uncommon in LMICs.[17] One site in Nigeria reported that these injuries were largely intentional (96%) with a male predominance. The investigators also noted that the upper extremity was most commonly injured. Of the total injuries, 19.2% of patients suffered open fractures and an equal number of tendon injuries. Peripheral nerve injury was identified in 8.1% of patients. The complication rate was noted to be high at 26%, with peripheral nerve deficits and wound infection the most common. Patients also were found to self-discharge prior to tendon and nerve repair, citing financial constraints.[17] Another study in rural South Africa echoed the high incidence of machete injury; 96% of patients had tendon injuries, with an average number of 4 tendons injured per patient. It is estimated that 44.9% of patients sustained peripheral nerve injuries, whereas 18% of patients had open fractures.[18]

Amputation of the upper extremity is another problem encountered in LMICs. Few data exist to determine the actual incidence of amputation of the upper extremity. One teaching hospital in Nigeria reported 58 traumatic amputations over a 10-year period.[19] A majority of these injuries were the result from traffic accidents in young men. In an Ethiopian university hospital, 31% of patients presenting for hand trauma involved digital amputations.[11] A majority of these cases were classified as minor (45.8%), whereas 17.8% of patients were classified as severe. Severe cases of amputation were caused by work-related interactions with machinery.[11]

Burn injury represents another category of hand trauma that a hand surgeon must master in LMICs. Worldwide, burns account for 7.1 million injuries each year, with the overwhelming majority occurring in LMICs (90%).[20] It also is estimated that more than 90% of burn-related deaths occur in LMICs.[21] A systematic review of the epidemiology of burn injuries sustained in Africa revealed that children younger than 5 years of age are at greatest risk for burn injury.[20] These burn injuries involved flame and hot liquids, with the most common place of injury within the home. This review also identified the upper extremity as the most common location for burn injuries in Africa.[20] A separate review also identified burn injury as the major cause of pediatric hand trauma (50%), followed by traffic accidents (37.5%) and occupational injuries (37.5%).[5]

GLOBAL SURGERY NEEDS

The worldwide disease burden is estimated to be surgical in nature in 11% to 32% of cases.[1,3] This percentage translates into 5 billion individuals who do not have access to safe and affordable surgery and anesthesia.[1] The poorest one-third of the world's population underwent only 2.5% of worldwide operations. Initial delays are encountered in seeking care, a result of financial, geographic, cultural, and educational reasons. Further delays in care result from an inability to reach hospitals owing to inadequate transportation. The final delay in surgical care results within the hospital, where arrival does not guarantee treatment.[1] In Uganda, for example, there is only 1 surgeon per 100,000 people, and 17 credentialed anesthesiologists in the country.[22] Patients travel an average of 68 km to the nearest referral hospital. The exact number of patients who are unable to present to a treatment facility is unknown.[22] The greatest surgical need is demonstrated in western sub-Saharan Africa, central sub-Saharan Africa, and eastern sub-Saharan Africa.[23] Macroeconomic implications from failure to adequately address the global burden of surgical disease are significant. Attributable losses of up to 1.25% of GDP or $20.7 trillion are estimated worldwide between 2015 and 2030.[24] The greatest economic losses are seen in LMICs.[24]

In 2015, the *Lancet* Commission on Global Surgery called for an up-scaling of cost-effective efforts in LMICs to overcome this global disease burden.[1] It was made clear that surgery is an "indivisible, indispensable part of healthcare." The Commission noted that investment in surgery and anesthesia capacity is affordable and life-saving and has a positive impact on the global economy.[1] The Commission proposed expansion of "coordinated, demand-driven international surgical support" to combat the inadequate infrastructure, medicine, equipment, finances, and human resources in LMICs.[1,22] It is this calling that drives the development of local surgical capacity, in which teaching hand surgery is an integral component.

CHALLENGES OF LATE PRESENTATION OF HAND PROBLEMS

The imbalance of a large burden of hand disease and inadequate surgical capacity results in limited or absent access to care. As a result, a majority of patients suffer from advanced disease conditions.[25] Pathology in LMICs differs greatly from that encountered in routine practice in HICs.[16] Surgical cases in LMICs also can be complicated

as a result of concomitant diseases, such as human immunodeficiency virus, tuberculosis, malaria, and leprosy.[25] Furthermore, diagnostic tools, such as nerve conduction studies, magnetic resonance imaging, computed tomography, and even plain radiographs, that are standard in HICs may not be available.[16]

Initial barriers to burn treatment in LMICs include poor transportation systems and lengthy distance of travel to centers capable of treating burn injury.[21] Furthermore, centers in LMICs often are ill equipped, with limited operating rooms, as well as shortages of blood, fluids, and medication.[21] The inability to provide safe anesthesia is yet another challenge. Most LMIC centers that treat burn patients are capable of performing acute burn resuscitation.[21] They often are not equipped to handle later stages of management, such as considerations for excision, skin grafting, and proper splinting. This environment results in wound healing by secondary intention and complications of wound infection and burn scar contracture.[10] The expertise for flap-based reconstruction often is lacking and leaving contractures untreated.[6] Even in hospitals where plastic surgery expertise is available, clinically significant limitations to treatment exist.

A needs assessment study was performed in a Mozambique hospital that is staffed with a team of plastic surgeons.[26] A majority of admitted patients suffered burn injuries with a predominance of upper extremity involvement. Mean time to skin grafting in burn patients was 53 days. The authors cited insufficient operating room block time, equipment limitations, and delays in medical optimization of patients as causes for delays in surgical care. These delays contributed to increased infection and contracture rates despite the availability of a plastic surgery team on staff.[26]

Delays in care also are seen in cases of amputation. At one Nigerian hospital, the average presentation of patients with upper extremity amputation was 98.9 hours after injury.[19] It was not surprising that 81% of patients presenting more than 24 hours after injury had wound infections after closure.[19] Deficiencies in triage and care of amputated parts also were noted.[19] Such delays and suboptimal treatment of amputated parts are barriers to replantation success.

Late presentation also is a challenge in the management of peripheral nerve injury. A retrospective case review of peripheral nerve injury in Brazil identified only 57.1% of patients presenting for electromyographic evaluation within 6 months after injury. The majority of these injuries involved upper extremity trauma.[27] This leaves a large proportion of patients presenting in a delayed fashion, which presents challenges to the possibility of surgical reinnervation. Similar delays were seen in a study from South Africa investigating the outcomes of end-to-side nerve transfer for nerve injury in the upper extremity. Here, patients had a median presentation from injury of 195 days with a range of 2 days to 455 days.[28] None of these patients demonstrated evidence of motor recovery postoperatively. The investigators identified delayed presentation and target muscle denervation atrophy as explanations for poor outcome.[28]

Congenital hand problems also frequently are seen in a delayed fashion. In Egypt, the mean age of presentation of congenital hand problems was 6 years old, with an age range from 2 months to 37 years of age.[29] This time frame contradicts the general timeline of performing congenital hand surgeries at 1 year to 2 years of age.[29] Thus, congenital hand problems present at a less desirable time period for surgery. The overwhelming conclusion is that hand surgery problems in the developing world are different from those in HICs. Surgeon-educators need to be aware of this difference.

PRINCIPLES OF AN EFFECTIVE EDUCATION PROGRAM

As the Lancet Commission has declared, an upscaling of efforts to build surgical capacity in LMICs is necessary. Surgeons in LMICs must be educated and supported through an effective long-term education program. The authors propose 5 principles that should govern an effective education program.

The first principle is that the most experienced teachers should teach in the developing world. Educating local surgeons in LMICs is challenging given the diverse and advanced pathology, the lack of perioperative resources, and the lack of local expert faculty and training opportunities.[15] To answer this call, the world's best teachers in a specific area of reconstructive surgery are needed. A surgeon operating and teaching outside the usual scope of practice has the potential to impart negative influences on local surgeons and patients. This is particularly true in light of the 20% higher complication rates of procedures performed in LMICs than those performed in HIC.[16,30] The developing world deserves educators with proved surgical skill sets and ability to teach.[3,6] These educators may be from both the developed world and the developing world.

A second principle of an effective education program is that perioperative safety should be modeled. Given the increase in complications in the perioperative setting of LMICs, it is important that an education program follows current OR safety culture in HICs. One observational study at a tertiary center in Ghana demonstrated a 0.65% perioperative mortality rate, or 1 death per 154 anesthetics.[31] In this case, 99% of deaths occurred in the postanesthesia care unit (PACU). This number contrasts with the standard anesthesia-related perioperative mortality rate of 1 death per 47,800 discharges.[31,32] Possible contributing factors included inconsistent physician oversight of hospital personnel, no physician involvement in PACUs, and a lack of specialized training for PACU nurses.[31] The investigators suggested that improvements in safety can be made through increased physician oversight, maintenance of operational ventilators, improved oxygen supply, availability of vital sign monitors, and improved outcomes reporting.[31]

Simple interventions, such as a surgical safety checklist, have also demonstrated improvement in perioperative safety. Haynes and colleagues[33] demonstrated that the utilization of a checklist based on the first edition of the World Health Organization Surgical Safety Checklist in hospitals of LMICs is feasible. Their prospective study resulted in a decrease in overall perioperative complication rate (11.7% to 6.8%; $P<.001$), including a decrease in the mortality rate (2.1% to 1.0%; $P = .006$) at these sites. The investigators reported that the checklist resulted in systems and behavioral changes by the surgical teams. The safety culture experienced in HICs, if used as a model for safety in LMICs, can improve on the quality of surgical capacity.

The third principle of an effective education program is that the same level of care should be taught overseas. Equal level of care applies not only to surgical management but also to anesthesia, antisepsis, and therapy. Operative indications and postoperative management also must be detailed and conveyed through LMIC cultural standards.[5] In addition to surgical capability, supporting infrastructure must be in place to support surgeons, such as reliable blood reserves, oxygen sources, pulse oximeters, and essential medications.[22] Unique in the treatment of hand surgery is the role of the hand therapist to ensure proper rehabilitation and optimal outcomes.[16] This critical team member needs to be included in efforts to teach hand surgery. The measurement of outcomes, including patient-reported outcomes, also is necessary for an effective education program.[34]

The fourth principle of an effective education program is sustainability. The traditional model of the surgical mission trip, which brings surgical services to LMIC in the short term, has fallen out of favor.[30] These strategies should be implemented only at locations where there are no alternative platforms.[30] Sustainability takes multiple forms, including funding, local surgeon education, ancillary staff education, and tracking of outcomes.[35] In addition, a needs assessment of LMIC institutions must be carried out to focus resources on high-impact areas of need.[4] LMIC partner institutions have differences in language, culture, clinical practice, and teaching curricula, which must be recognized.[4] Sustainable efforts should consist of a collaborative relationship, where roles and expectations of all parties are clearly defined.[4,5]

The Massachusetts General Hospital (MGH) Global Surgery Initiative (GSI) is one example of the successful implementation of a sustainable collaboration.[36] MGH GSI created a long-term partnership in an LMIC setting. An ideal partnership was found with the Mbarara University of Science and Technology of Uganda, an academic center with an existing medical school, nursing school, desire to expand surgical capability, and interest in research. The investigators suggested that such a model can be duplicated in the establishment of other academic global surgery programs.[36] In another example, Smith and colleagues[37] demonstrated that a long-term outreach program in the treatment of chronic suppurative otitis media resulted in the ability of local surgeons to safely and confidently perform tympanoplasty, mastoidectomy, and ossiculoplasty. Training fellows from an HIC were deployed to Cambodia for a 4-month to 6-month residency to deliver in-country training to local surgeons. The investigators reported that surgeons trained through the program were able to perform these procedures independently and increase operative volume. Moreover, additional trainees are being taught by the local team.[37] Such a model offers sustainability in the development of surgical capacity in LMIC.

The fifth and final principle of an effective education program is the identification, tracking, and certification of trainees. In LMICs, there often are few positions for specialty-specific surgical training available to recent medical graduates.[6] Each additional surgeon trained likely will have a positive impact on the treatment of surgical disease in LMICs.[25] Trainees should be identified, tracked, and certified. This formal process imparts appropriate attention and resources to be provided to individual trainees. Most importantly, tracking and certification will ensure competency of newly trained hand surgeons.

COMPONENTS OF A GLOBAL HAND SURGERY CURRICULUM

A specialized curriculum aimed at teaching hand surgery in developing countries must be designed. The authors suggest 5 important components of a global hand surgery curriculum. The first component includes expert faculty. Needs in developing surgical capacity are not defined simply by costs of equipment; rather, they are medical knowledge, surgical skills, and dedicated doctors.[1] Expert faculty from HICs should be utilized to meet these needs because they can provide support in the form of financial, teaching, and assessment resources. Remote contributions also are possible through innovation in telemedicine, online learning, and simulation.[4] The emergence of global surgery as a viable academic pathway helps foster those interested in leading long-term global surgery efforts.[3] Kristhnaswami and colleagues have discussed a framework for developing such a field. An academic global surgeon would seek to incorporate academic surgery values of education, clinical service, scholarship, and advocacy.[3] These values follow the *Lancet* Commission's call to improve surgical care in LMICs. These surgeons would develop sustained collaborations in research, education, and training with colleagues from LMICs. Currently, only 30% of academic institutions have such long-term partnerships. A major focus of an academic global surgery position is developing the best method of training surgeons in LMICs. Such efforts include remote learning capabilities, such as online curricula and virtual simulation. In addition, attention to surgical innovation and advocacy add to the construct of the academic global surgery faculty.[3]

The second component is a competency-based curriculum. A global surgery curriculum should focus on goal state performance, model application of learned material in patient care, be defined in measurable behaviors, and clearly outline expectations of trainees.[38,39] The focus should not be on the number of surgical procedures; rather, attention should be paid to identifying procedures with the greatest educational value.[6] A curriculum must not focus solely on the technical aspects of an operation. Educators should detail operative indications as well as postoperative management. Furthermore, careful attention to local cultural norms is necessary.[6]

Shaye and colleagues[38] developed a competency-based curriculum for facial trauma in an LMIC setting. The authors utilized a backward planning strategy, which resulted in a successful curriculum implementation with positive educational outcomes. Such a method of curriculum development first identifies common and specific clinical problems. Subsequently, educators proceed to reverse engineer the knowledge and skill sets needed to treat each problem. The investigators developed a curriculum on facial trauma by focusing on the top patient problems presenting in the LMIC setting: (1) acute airway and bleeding; (2) blindness, orbital hematoma, and zygomaticomaxillary complex fracture; (3) mandible fractures, Le Fort fractures, and dental occlusion; and, finally, (4) wound care principles and laceration repair.[38] The investigators then identified performance and competencies that a surgeon requires to effectively treat each case. In an LMIC setting, educational goals need to be strategic and include not only medical knowledge and surgical skills but also nontechnical skills and attitudes.[38] Thus, with the goal of an independent surgeon in mind, end competencies of knowledge, skills, and attitudes can be taught through lecture, discussion, and exercise.[38]

The third component of a global hand surgery curriculum is a milestone measurement tool. This strategy is modeled after the Accreditation Council for Graduate Medical Education (ACGME), the accreditation organization for graduate medical training in the United States. Milestones across the core competencies of medical knowledge, patient care, interpersonal and communication skills, professionalism, practice-based learning and improvement, and systems-based practice are evaluated throughout training.[40] The ACGME milestones for plastic surgery residents can be adapted to suit the appropriate skill sets in LMICs.[41] These metrics will serve not only to assess the trainee but also to evaluate the training program itself.[4] Other measures that should be tracked are the number of trainees, quality of clinical outcomes, and examination scores.[4] The use of a milestone measurement tool in LMICs ensures the same high standards of surgical training in HICs.

The fourth component of a global surgery curriculum consists of hands-on training. Intraoperative teaching allows for careful observation and real-time feedback by expert surgeons.[41] Expert hand surgery educators have demonstrated that new techniques, such as the pedicled groin flap, ligament rebalancing, and Z-plasty, are readily learned by local surgeons in LMICs. On follow-up trips, local surgeons continued to use these previously introduced techniques.[6] Hands-on training also should include teaching through cost-effective simulation. For example, the implementation of an end-ileostomy model in Rwanda demonstrated sustained skill improvements for trainees in both HICs and LMICs.[42] Advances in wearable technology also can facilitate hands-on training through teleproctoring.[43] McCullough and colleagues[43] demonstrated that the use of Google Glass enabled the successful teleproctoring of 12 reconstructive hand surgeries in Mozambique. The wearable Google Glass device was used to stream live video from the Mozambique surgeon's field of vision while projecting overlaid images

remotely generated from the expert surgeon in the United States. The authors reported that the teleproctoring allowed the field surgeon to successfully perform unfamiliar rotational and pedicle flaps procedures without complication. Both the field surgeon and proctoring surgeon found the device useful in teaching hand surgery in the preoperative and intraoperative settings.[43]

Digital training makes up the fifth component of a successful global hand surgery curriculum. Digital simulation, although mostly utilized by training centers in HICs, also is beneficial in LMICs.[42] Plana and colleagues[44] demonstrated the success of a virtual surgical simulator for cleft lip and palate repair in LMICs. The simulator included modules on anatomy, surgical marking, and operative technique with intraoperative footage; 70% of countries accessing the simulator were LMICs. The investigators emphasized their online simulator contributed to sustainable capacity building through digital training.[44] In Rwanda, the Touch Surgery smartphone application that provides step-by-step instruction in operative technique was used. Use of the application resulted in improved technical skills in tendon repair compared with traditional textbook-based learning.[45] Another example of a digital training platform is the International Microsurgery Club Facebook group. This group fosters international collaboration and case discussion through social media.[46] Such a platform should be highlighted in the LMIC setting, where surgical consultants often are absent. The use of digital training in LMICs may help address the lack of local surgeon faculty and training opportunities.

The final component of a global hand surgery curriculum is certification. As discussed previously, an effective curriculum must include a milestones measurement tool. As trainees in LMICs gain experience, objective evaluations of their competency can be made over time. Trainees with advanced skills can then be identified and certified as competent. This certification is the ultimate goal of establishing increased surgical capacity through education. Certification for trainees will ensure underserved patients in LMICs will be treated appropriately by newly trained local surgeons.[41] It also will ensure responsible investment into local surgical capacity, where resources and support can be directed to certified surgeons. It is critical that programs from HICs collaborate effectively with local certifying bodies.

RESURGE INTERNATIONAL GLOBAL TRAINING PROGRAM

ReSurge International is a nongovernmental, nonprofit organization based in the United States that delivers reconstructive surgery to underserved populations in LMICs. A major focus of ReSurge International is building local surgical capacity.[41] The ReSurge global training program (RGTP) embodies the principles of an effective education program with a curriculum designed for teaching reconstructive surgery in LMICs.[41] The RGTP curriculum features a digital library of lectures developed by expert surgeon faculty. These lectures are easily accessible and free to access for trainees in LMICs. For example, "Congenital Hand" and "Hand Trauma" are 2 of the 60 lectures that make up the collection.

The ReSurge visiting educator trip is another important component of the RGTP. The visiting educator trip consists of 1 to 2 expert reconstructive surgeons (board certified), an anesthesiologist, a therapist, a nurse, and, at times, a pediatrician. These team members engage in direct teaching with their host institution counterparts. This setting results in a concentrated hands-on apprenticeship style of teaching. Local surgeons and trainees also are evaluated by the visiting educators using a standardized milestones metric.[41] This evaluation tool is modeled after the ACGME milestones.[41] Visiting educator trips occur in the context of long-term collaboration between ReSurge and LMIC partner sites. In this manner, the same trainees are identified, educated, and evaluated over time.

A retrospective review by Sue and colleagues[41] demonstrated that this competency-based curriculum resulted in the evaluation of 149 trainees in LMICs. Furthermore, these trainees displayed improved milestone scores over time.[41] As surgical competency increases, trainees reach a level where they are selected to become outreach partners. As an outreach partner, surgeons are able to be reimbursed per qualifying reconstructive procedure to encourage reconstructive efforts in underserved populations.[41]

The RGTP also features the use of readily accessible technologies for surgical training. The RGTP surveyed its community of expert surgeon faculty, outreach partners, and trainees on the use of social media for surgical education (Deptula P, RGTP Facebook group, unpublished data, 2019). International outreach partners and trainees from LMICs demonstrated overwhelmingly favorable attitudes toward the use social media in surgical education. The RGTP Facebook group was created as a result of this demand. This closed online community of surgeon experts and international trainees offers an easily accessible educational resource using the ubiquitous social media platform. The RGTP features the library of RGTP lectures posted to the group. The group also enables a course tracking tool to monitor the progress of trainees as they work through the lectures. It also serves as an immediate means to share difficult cases and receive real-time expert feedback. In this manner, surgeons working in resource-poor regions have access to world expert opinion. The authors reported a successful launch of the Facebook group and early successes since the group's creation in November 2018 (Deptula P, RGTP Facebook group, unpublished data, 2019). As the RGTP Facebook group continues to develop, future initiatives will include hosting live video lectures, a formal mentorship program, and research collaborations.

SUMMARY

Efforts to bolster hand surgery capacity in the developing world are needed to address the global burden of surgical disease. By teaching hand surgery in LMICs, access to hand surgery can be improved worldwide. Hand surgery in the developing world is unique and requires an effective teaching strategy. Principles to guide the education of hand surgeons in LMICs include employing the best teachers in the world, modeling HIC operating room safety culture, teaching equivalent level of care in LMICs, attention to sustainability, and identification and certification of trainees. Components of an effective hand surgery curriculum include expert surgeon faculty, a competency-based curriculum, a milestone assessment tool, hands-on training, digital training, and certification RGTP is one example of many new programs that share principles and components of an effective hand surgery curriculum for the developing world. Despite challenges, such initiatives must be continued and supported by the community of hand surgeons.

REFERENCES

1. Meara JG, Leather AJM, Hagander L, et al. Global Surgery 2030: evidence and solutions for achieving health, welfare, and economic development. Lancet 2015;386(9993):569–624.

2. Alkire BC, Raykar NP, Shrime MG, et al. Global access to surgical care: a modelling study. Lancet Glob Health 2015;3(6):e316–23.

3. Krishnaswami S, Stephens CQ, Yang GP, et al. An academic career in global surgery: a position paper from the Society of University Surgeons Committee on Academic Global Surgery. Surgery 2018;163(4):954–60.

4. Rickard J, Ntirenganya F, Ntakiyiruta G, et al. Global health in the 21st century: equity in surgical training partnerships. J Surg Educ 2019;76(1):9–13.

5. Chung KY, Hanemaayer A, Poenaru D. Pediatric hand surgery in global health: the role for international outreach. Ann Plast Surg 2017;78(2):162–70.

6. Chung KC, Kotsis SV. Teaching pediatric hand surgery in vietnam. Hand (N Y) 2007;2(1):16–24.

7. Goldfarb CA. Congenital hand anomalies: a review of the literature, 2009–2012. J Hand Surg 2013; 38(9):1854–9.

8. Dy CJ, Swarup I, Daluiski A. Embryology, diagnosis, and evaluation of congenital hand anomalies. Curr Rev Musculoskelet Med 2014;7(1):60–7.

9. Siotos C, Ibrahim Z, Bai J, et al. Hand injuries in low- and middle-income countries: systematic review of existing literature and call for greater attention. Public Health 2018;162:135–46.

10. Semer NB, Sullivan SR, Meara JG. Plastic surgery and global health: How plastic surgery impacts the global burden of surgical disease. J Plast Reconstr Aesthet Surg 2010;63(8):1244–8.

11. Ahmed E. The management outcome of acute hand injury in Tikur Anbessa University Hospital, Addis Ababa, Ethiopia. East Cent Afr J Surg 2010;15(1): 48–56.

12. Ihekire O, Salawu SAI, Opadele T. Causes of hand injuries in a developing country. Can J Surg 2010; 53(3):161–6.

13. Al-Husuny A, Rampal L, Manohar A, et al. Work-related hand injuries: type, location, cause, mechanism and severity in a tertiary hospital. MJMHS 2012;8(2):41–9.

14. Sabitu K, Iliyasu Z, Dauda MM. Awareness of occupational hazards and utilization of safety measures among welders in Kaduna metropolis, northern Nigeria. Ann Afr Med 2009;8(1):46–51.

15. Kaisha WO, Khainga S. Causes and pattern of unilateral hand injuries. East Afr Med J 2008;85(3): 123–8.

16. Nugent AG, Panthaki Z, Thaller S. The planning and execution of surgical hand mission trips in developing countries. J Craniofac Surg 2015;26(4): 1055–7.

17. Omoke NI, Madubueze CC. Machete injuries as seen in a Nigerian teaching hospital. Injury 2010; 41(1):120–4.

18. Howard N, Holmes WJM, Price CE, et al. Severity of upper-limb panga injuries and infection rates associated with early v. late tendon repair. S Afr J Surg 2014;52(1):22–5.

19. Omoke NI, Chukwu COO, Madubueze CC, et al. Traumatic extremity amputation in a Nigerian setting: patterns and challenges of care. Int Orthop 2012; 36(3):613–8.

20. Rybarczyk MM, Schafer JM, Elm CM, et al. A systematic review of burn injuries in low- and middle-income countries: epidemiology in the WHO-defined African Region. Afr J Emerg Med 2017;7(1):30–7.

21. Gupta S, Wong EG, Mahmood U, et al. Burn management capacity in low and middle-income countries: a systematic review of 458 hospitals across 14 countries. Int J Surg 2014;12(10):1070–3.

22. Linden AF, Sekidde FS, Galukande M, et al. Challenges of surgery in developing countries: a survey of surgical and anesthesia capacity in Uganda's Public Hospitals. World J Surg 2012; 36(5):1056–65.

23. Rose J, Weiser TG, Hider P, et al. Estimated need for surgery worldwide based on prevalence of diseases: a modelling strategy for the WHO Global Health Estimate. Lancet Glob Health 2015;3:S13–20.

24. Alkire BC, Shrime MG, Dare AJ, et al. Global economic consequences of selected surgical diseases: a modelling study. Lancet Glob Health 2015;3: S21–7.

25. Hayton RA, Donley DK, Fekadu A, et al. Surgical volunteerism as a collaborative teaching activity can benefit surgical residents in low-middle income countries. Int J Surg 2017;48:34–7.

26. Guzman KJ, Gemo N, Martins DB, et al. Current challenges of plastic surgical care in Sub-Saharan Africa (Maputo, Mozambique). Plast Reconstr Surg Glob Open 2018;6(8):e1893.

27. Kouyoumdjian JA, Graça CR, Ferreira VFM. A retrospective survey of 1124 cases. Neurol India 2017;65(3):551–5.

28. Pienaar C, Swan MC, De Jager W, et al. Clinical experience with end-to-side nerve transfer. J Hand Surg 2004;29(5):438–43.

29. Abulezz T, Talaat M, Elsani A, et al. Congenital hand anomalies in Upper Egypt. Indian J Plast Surg 2016; 49(2):206–13.

30. Shrime MG, Sleemi A, Ravilla TD. Charitable platforms in global surgery: a systematic review of their effectiveness, cost-effectiveness, sustainability, and role training. World J Surg 2015;39(1):10–20.

31. Brouillette MA, Aidoo AJ, Hondras MA, et al. Anesthesia capacity in ghana: a teaching hospital's resources, and the national workforce and education. Anesth Analg 2017;125(6):2063–71.

32. Li G, Warner M, Lang BH, et al. Epidemiology of anesthesia-related mortality in the United States, 1999-2005. Anesthesiology 2009;110(4):759–65.

33. Haynes AB, Weiser TG, Berry WR, et al. A surgical safety checklist to reduce morbidity and mortality in a global population. N Engl J Med 2009;360(5): 491–9.

34. Giladi AM, McGlinn EP, Shauver MJ, et al. Measuring outcomes and determining long-term disability after revision amputation for treatment of traumatic finger and thumb amputation injuries. Plast Reconstr Surg 2014;134(5):746e–55e.

35. Zender CA, Clancy K, Thuener JE, et al. Surgical outreach and microvascular surgery in developing countries. Oral Oncol 2018;81:69–74.

36. Chao TE, Riesel JN, Anderson GA, et al. Building a global surgery initiative through evaluation, collaboration, and training: the Massachusetts general hospital experience. J Surg Educ 2015;72(4):e21–8.

37. Smith AKK, Sokdavy T, Sothea C, et al. Implementation and results of a surgical training programme for chronic suppurative otitis media in Cambodia. J Laryngol Otol 2018;132(08):711–7.

38. Shaye DA, Tollefson T, Shah I, et al. Backward planning a Craniomaxillofacial trauma curriculum for the surgical Workforce in low-resource settings. World J Surg 2018;42(11):3514–9.

39. Albanese MA, Mejicano G, Mullan P, et al. Defining characteristics of educational competencies. Med Educ 2008;42(3):248–55.

40. 100 years of surgical education: The past, present, and future. The Bulletin 2013. Available at: http://bulletin.facs.org/2013/07/100-years-of-surgical-education/. Accessed November 2, 2018.

41. Sue GR, Covington WC, Chang J. The ReSurge global training program: a model for surgical training and capacity building in global reconstructive surgery. Ann Plast Surg 2018;81(3):250–6.

42. Tansley G, Bailey JG, Gu Y, et al. Efficacy of surgical simulation training in a low-income country. World J Surg 2016;40(11):2643–9.

43. McCullough MC, Kulber L, Sammons P, et al. Google glass for remote surgical tele-proctoring in low- and middle-income countries: a feasibility study from Mozambique. Plast Reconstr Surg Glob Open 2018;6:e1999.

44. Plana NM, Diaz-Siso JR, Culnan DM, et al. The first year of global cleft surgery education through digital simulation: a proof of concept. Cleft Palate Craniofac J 2018;55(4):626–9.

45. Bunogerane GJ, Taylor K, Lin Y, et al. Using touch surgery to improve surgical education in low- and middle-income settings: a randomized control trial. J Surg Educ 2018;75(1):231–7.

46. Chang TN-J, Hsieh F, Wang Z-T, et al. Social media mediate the education of the global microsurgeons: the experience from International Microsurgery Club. Microsurgery 2018;38(5):596–7.

Ethics in Global Surgery

Nnenaya Agochukwu-Mmonu, MD, MS[a,b,*], Kevin C. Chung, MD, MS[c]

KEYWORDS

- Global surgery • Ethics • Medical ethics • Low- and middle-income countries

KEY POINTS

- Autonomy, beneficence, nonmaleficence, and justice are central ethical principles that are essential to the delivery of surgical services globally.
- Although cultural and language barriers can make following these basic ethical principles challenging, it is important that concerted effort is made to follow these principles and establish trust between surgeons and patients.
- The *body count mentality*, aiming to complete as many cases as possible, which is prevalent in short-term medical mission trips, must be abandoned to ensure delivery of high-quality surgical services in low-income and middle-income countries.

INTRODUCTION

One-third of the global burden of disease encompasses surgery.[1] One-third of the world's population lives in low and middle-income countries. As the population grows and longevity increases in the world's poorest countries, the need for surgical services is estimated to increase by insurmountable proportions. In fact, it is estimated that 143 million additional surgical procedures will be needed in low and middle-income countries.[2] Furthermore, it is estimated that 1.4 million deaths could be avoided yearly with basic surgical procedures.[3] The Lancet Global Surgery commission released a report, "Global Surgery 2030," which highlights that the poorest sector of the population receives 3.5% of all surgical procedures.[1–4] Reasons for this disparity are numerous and include poverty, physician shortages, and infrastructural challenges. To combat this disparity, short-term surgical missions (STSMs) have increased, led by

nongovernmental organizations, private organizations, and academic institutions with the goal of providing much-needed surgical care. This is especially true for hand surgery, given the direct link of hand injuries and/or anomalies to productivity.[5] In the provision of this much-needed surgical care, however, it is important that ethical principles are followed.

In the recent decades, much effort has gone into protection strategies for research subjects, given the potential exploitative nature of research.[6] These same protections for patients who are cared for as part of humanitarian missions are largely nonexistent, despite that humanitarian missions can also be an unequal relationship. In 1997, the Institute of Medicine published a report on "America's vital interest in global health."[7] This report states that, "America has a vital and direct stake in the health of people around the globe, and this interest derives from both America's long and enduring tradition of humanitarian concern and

Disclosure Statement: Research reported in this publication was supported in part from a Midcareer Investigator Award in Patient-Oriented Research (2K24 AR053120-06 to Dr K.C. Chung) and University of Michigan Global REACH.

a Department of Urology, The University of Michigan Medical School, University of Michigan, 2800 Plymouth Road, Building 14, Room G100-19, Ann Arbor, MI 48109, USA; b Department of Urology, University of California, San Francisco, 1001 Potrero Avenue, Building 5, Room 3A16, San Francisco, CA 94110, USA; c Section of Plastic Surgery, The University of Michigan Medical School, University of Michigan Health System, 2130 Taubman Center, SPC 5340, 1500 East Medical Center Drive, Ann Arbor, MI 48109-5340, USA
* Corresponding author. Department of Urology, University of California, San Francisco, 1001 Potrero Avenue, Building 5, Room 3A16, San Francisco, CA 94110.
E-mail address: agochukw@umich.edu

Hand Clin 35 (2019) 421–427
https://doi.org/10.1016/j.hcl.2019.07.013

compelling reasons of enlightened self-interest." Although these concerns are evident in the commitment of America to the well-being of the world, this same stake in the health of people and self-interest must be rooted in ethical guidelines.

In the pursuit of this well-being, especially for the most vulnerable, we must hold ourselves to the same standards as we would if we were treating a family member and not betray the trust that patients place in us. Practice patterns should be universally applicable and based on a standard set of ethical guidelines, as opposed to conforming to what is perceived as acceptable in a certain setting. The avoidance of exploitative and imperialistic practices in the delivery of health care worldwide, especially in humanitarian missions, is essential. In this review, we discuss ethical principles, including autonomy, beneficence, nonmaleficence, and justice[8] as they pertain to the delivery of surgical care on STSMs and global surgery.

Autonomy

The ethics principle of autonomy states that patients have the right to choose or refuse treatment based on informed consent.[9] They should be informed of the risks, benefits, and alternatives to treatment and no treatment. Respecting the autonomy of an individual means that patients are to be consulted to ensure they agree, before a procedure is done. Moreover, it requires that we do not deceive patients.[10] If patients do not understand explanations about their illness, every effort should be made to inform them. In low-resource settings, communication barriers and cultural aspects may impair this informed consent process. In addition, patients also may traditionally have no say in their care. The ultimate decision for treatment may be from the head of the family or a leader in the community. This may be amplified in medical mission trips, where patients may perceive foreign doctors as having authority. Difficulties in communication should not be an impediment to respect for autonomy, but rather, should be a reason to make a directed effort to effectively communicate and ensure there is comprehension.

A theoretic example of this in medical missions is a surgical team of hand surgeons, including medical students, residents, and attendings, goes to a low-resource country to perform surgeries for congenital hand deformities for a 3-week period. Before arriving, there is brief communication with the local surgeons and the local surgeons inform the visiting surgeons on the cases. The local surgeons gather patients for the operations and when the surgical team arrives, there are 100 patients waiting in line. There is no interpreter except for the operating room nurse who is also busy with other tasks. After each patient is examined, the surgical team decides the operating plan as the patient is induced and prepared for surgery. The surgical team does not explain to the patients what they plan to do, and the patient is unaware of the risks, benefits, and alternatives to the procedure. They have been told only that they need the procedure and many of them have had these ailments for many years. In addition, the patient is unaware of everyone on the teams' respective roles. Each day the surgical team sets out to the operating room and patients are brought in, there is little to no communication between patients and the surgical team. This continues until the end of 3 weeks, at which point the surgical team leaves the site. There is no record of the procedures. In addition, many pictures of the patients are taken throughout the trip, without consent.

There are a few ethical issues in this scenario that arise from communication and cultural barriers. Cultural differences have a high propensity to result in an environment where expectations, values, and an attempt at shared decision-making are abandoned. In this case, the patients do not know what exact procedure is to be done, nor have they been informed of the risks, benefits, and alternatives of said procedures by the surgical team. This would be unacceptable in the operating surgeon's home-based hospital and may even lead to revocation of a license to practice. In addition, the patients are not aware that trainees (medical students and residents) are involved in their care. Trainees are increasingly engaging in short-term medical mission trips. According to the Association of American Medical Colleges, 30% of medical students participated in a global health volunteer experience during medical school.[11] A survey of the American College of Surgeons demonstrated that 92% of residents were interested in international electives.[12] There is also debate that operations done during an international mission should potentially count toward case requirements set by the Accreditation Council for Graduate Medical Education, especially for programs that may fall below national averages.[13] Although this is an educational opportunity, which can greatly impact trainees by teaching them about the importance of fiscal awareness, cost savings, patient management, and cultural sensitivity, it is not an opportunity for trainees to practice in a capacity that would be impermissible otherwise. In addition, more time and energy should be spent sharing skills and techniques with local surgeons. Trainees also often gain first-hand experience in brief periods of time that they otherwise would not receive at their institutions.[14] This may lead to a scenario in which trainees may be operating at a capacity that would not be permitted at their home institutions. In fact, during surgical missions, residents may perform 25 cases in 5 to 7 days.[13] Trainees must have clear roles and limitations set by both host and visiting institutions.[15]

Another positive aspect of international missions is that trainees may feel a heightened sense of responsibility for surgery in low-resource settings.[16,17] It is crucial that this sense of responsibility is not misplaced and that trainees be held to the same or even higher standards on an international surgical mission as they would be at their home institution. The Working Group on Ethics Guidelines for Global Health Training (WEIGHT) developed guidelines for trainees to avoid ethical breaches.[18] They specifically recommend adequate mentorship and supervision and provide framework for strengthening global health partnerships. In essence, before a medical student has sworn the Hippocratic oath, he or she cannot operate on patients in an impermissible capacity with little to no supervision. Individuals, including trainees and their supervisors, may feel performing at a level that is beyond their expertise is justified based on resource limitations and the lack of other options for the vulnerable populations they encounter. However, even if patients have limited or no access to surgery because of surgeon shortages or excessive costs of care, it is unethical to perform in a capacity that one does not typically perform and/or is unprepared. In addition, trainees may experience stress and guilt from this, as well as place themselves at unacceptable risks.[19] DeCamp and colleagues[20] established ethics curriculums for short-term global health trainees that aims to increase awareness of ethical issues in global health. There is evidence that in-country trainees also question the ethics of visiting surgeons. A study on perspectives from trainees in Uganda revealed that 31% of trainees were uncomfortable with ethics of some clinical decisions made by visiting faculty, and 40% felt international groups had a neutral or negative impact on patient care.[21]

These principles also apply to practicing surgeons operating in a capacity for which they are unprepared. For example, a surgeon who does not do cleft lips in his or her practice may feel justified to do these surgeries in low-resource settings. Despite the lack of subspecialty training, one may again have the perception that someone doing something is better than no one doing anything,

given the poor access and physician shortages in low-resource settings. There is no process of certification or verification of licenses for STSM trips. Until there is an established system of central reporting and certification, a common moral language, specifically abidance with the Hippocratic oath, is necessary. This is a complex situation because patients may perceive a better outcome if they receive surgeries from surgeons abroad due to poor confidence in the local health care system.[22] It is important that despite this belief, and that the surgical team has come from abroad, that one does not take advantage of these vulnerable populations.

Although other often-cited advantages in international surgical missions do exist, such as the opportunity to treat patients with complex, advanced diseases, these conditions are also very rarely encountered in the United States and other settings abroad. This can pose a risk for the patient, as the surgeon is operating in an unfamiliar setting, with limited resources on unfamiliar conditions. Commonalities in developing nations, such as malnutrition,[23,24] endemic parasitic diseases,[25] and sickle cell trait or disease,[26] would pose a unique challenge for the visiting surgeon and one must recognize this and operate in one's capacity and purview. This cannot be done without proper planning and partnerships with local health care providers. A critical adage is that a surgeon should not perform an operation that he or she is uncomfortable doing and if the condition is not ideal. For example, if there is a lack of suitable microsurgical instruments, a free flap procedure must not be undertaken given it will incur a much greater risk of failure.

Although some patients in vulnerable populations may be culturally accustomed to a paternalistic system,[27] practitioners are obliged to adhere to a universal standard of practice and informed consent; in other words, the Hippocratic oath is universally applicable and should always be at the forefront of the surgical team's mission. The vulnerability of these individuals puts them at high risk of exploitation, and it is important to have increased sensitivity as we seek to do good. Medical missions, although largely well-intentioned, can easily fall victim to paternalism and result in negative, unintended consequences. By adhering to autonomy, we can ensure patients understand procedures they are to undergo and the role of everyone involved.

Beneficence and Nonmaleficence

Beneficence is to do good, whereas nonmaleficence is to do no harm.[8] These principles often work in parallel. It is worth mentioning that no surgeon sets out to intentionally do harm. The Hippocratic oath that physicians take on medical school completion explicitly states "first, do no harm." We are tasked to provide benefit with minimal harm. Physicians are automatically drawn to short-term missions.[28] This is evidenced by the growth of medical volunteerism that result in personal expenditures of up to $2 billion per year for individuals who engage in volunteerism.[29] Organizations that offer short-term mission trips have annual expenditures of $250 million.[30] Despite the altruism involved in medical volunteerism and medical mission trips, in the quest to do good and allow for equal access and care to individuals worldwide, especially in low-resource settings, harm often can be an unintended consequence.

An example of this is in the following scenario. On the same 3-week medical mission trip for congenital hand deformities, as is customary, the most complex cases are undertaken. This is problematic in considering the long-term ramifications and no plan in place for follow-up. There is no follow-up care provided by the operating surgeons and the home-based surgeons are unaware of both what complications to expect and what course of action to take for complications that develop. Moreover, certain complications may not be solvable depending on a country's resources. Accountability is compromised. Instead, the body count mentality prevails in which a team strives to do as many operations as possible, with little to no regard for outcomes.[31] This represents prioritization of quantity over quality.[32]

The pursuit of high-quality care is not limited to high-income countries. The global health quality revolution has recently come to the forefront.[33,34] It is estimated that 5.7 to 8.4 million deaths in low and middle-income countries are attributed to receiving poor-quality care[34]; 2.1 million of these deaths are attributed to deaths in the postoperative period.[35] It is estimated that this results in a subsequent loss of productivity of more than $1 trillion per year. To advance the current landscape to one in which safe, high-quality surgery becomes normative, the body count mentality must be abandoned. It is crucial that the same quality standards adhered to in home-based practices are followed in low-resource settings. With no accountability and follow-up, morbidity and mortality are unknown, and a well-intentioned STSM trip can result in an extra burden for the patient and health care system.

Another problem in the preceding scenario is that the surgical team is operating with limited resources, which has the potential to compromise the quality of an operation, as the surgical team is now operating in modified ways that are unfamiliar to them. The unintended consequence of harm prevails in a setting in which the goal is to do good. The solution, however, is not to add familiar health care equipment. Importantly, the World Health Organization supports this notion, and reports that if donations are made without planning and collaboration with the receiving health care system, these donations can be burdensome to the receiving health care system.[36] A volunteer surgeon must have sufficient skills to adapt to the limited resource setting and perhaps even learn from the local surgeons to make do with what they have, while achieving acceptable outcomes.

Many of these pitfalls and breaches of ethical guidelines on STSMs can be avoided by following the principles of beneficence and nonmaleficence. Several things can be done to avoid compromise of follow-up care. Integrating the home-based physicians as co-surgeons into the surgeries as they are done is essential. Often, visiting surgeons operate with their team, and the local surgeon does not scrub in. Establishing collaborations and partnerships allows for an exchange of ideas, levels the playing field, and creates a respectful environment in which everyone is seen as equally capable and responsible. Venturing into someone else's operating room, operating on their patients who have relinquished their trust into the surgeons, and taking an approach of believing he or she is superior because he or she has traveled from abroad is counterproductive and can lead to adverse patient outcomes. With collaboration, everyone can benefit; benefits include joint preoperative planning, the impartation of knowledge of procedures undertaken, including potential expectations and complications, and follow-up. The American Academy of Pediatrics Delivery of Surgical Care Subcommittee and the American Pediatric Surgical Association Global Pediatric Surgery Committee established consensus recommendations and guidelines for short-term missions to ensure they are ethical, safe, and responsible.[37] A key component of these guidelines includes planning, follow-up, and sustainability. In addition, the recommendations advise one to establish long-term relationships as part of these short-term trips.

Although record keeping can be challenging in low-resource settings, a concerted effort can be made to keep accurate records to ensure that patients receive appropriate follow-up and to safeguard that quality is not compromised. An open line of communication with the community and local physicians serves to anticipate complications and timely management. Finally, collaboration and establishment of long-term relationships with the local surgeons and health care team teaches the volunteer surgeon how to apply available in-country resources. A call for international morbidity and mortality conferences also has been proposed as a method of accountability.[38] An example of effective record keeping is from Operation Smile, in which an electronic medical record was established for evaluation of perioperative complications.[39]

An example of effective collaboration to follow outcomes is in a study by Johnston and colleagues,[40] which analyzed early outcomes of a humanitarian surgical organization that provided surgery on 6 STSMs to Sierra Leone and Ghana. In this study, of 372 surgeries done, there were 26 complications reported. Data collection was feasible, and partnerships with local health care providers was essential for preoperative and follow-up care. A study on operations carried out by a charitable organization based in Spain, Surgical Solidarity, evaluated the quality of hernia surgery in Cameroon and Mali.[41] The outcomes were compared with outcomes of hernia procedures in Spain by the Quality Control section of the Spanish Association of Surgeons. Short-term follow-up was done by the charitable organization and long-term follow-up was done at the next visit by the charitable organization. Local health officials revisited all cases at 6 and 12 months and communicated with the surgical team. Quality indicators, including morbidity and mortality, were collected. Sixty percent of patients were evaluated in follow-up by either the surgical team or local health care agents. Complication rates were similar in Spain, Cameroon, and Mali and with careful attention to detail, quality was not compromised. Follow-up, however, was noted to be problematic in Cameroon and Mali, which emphasizes the importance of involving local health care teams in follow-up.

Justice

Justice in medical health is fairness and includes 3 aspects: distributive justice, rights-based justice, and legal justice. Distributive justice relates to resource allocation and is especially important in low-resource settings. Rights-based justice is respect for an individual's rights. Legal justice is the respect for morally acceptable laws. As the imprint of STSMs increase, how does one ensure fair and culturally appropriate distribution of resources that are already limited? Should these resources instead go to conditions that affect more individuals, such as malnutrition, parasitic diseases, and human immunodeficiency virus/

AIDS? This is why for many years, surgery was regarded as the "neglected stepchild" in global health.[42] In resource-limited countries, the decision on provision of care for surgical ailments must be made while considering other needs in the country. STSM trips should not create a competition for resources that are already scarce.

For example, the previously described surgical team is operating in one operating room and has noticed that the power supply is not reliable. In addition, they are required to wait 3 hours between cases to allow for re-processing of instruments. They express frustration and decide that they will not return to this location. Surgeons involved in STSMs likely are exposed to working conditions of which they are unaccustomed. If every surgeon takes this approach of abandoning a mission because of unsuitable environments, then patients with surgical diseases will be neglected and nonmaleficence ensues. For example, the need for electricity could result in resource diversion from other needed areas, such as for incubators in the neonatal intensive care unit. One must respect the allocation of resources, which are already set. For example, a hospital that has 3 operating rooms has designated 1 operating room to be allocated for the short-term medical mission cases and another to be for routine cases that were scheduled 6 months in advance. The final operating room is on hold for emergencies. The surgeons on the mission trip decide that it would be best if they use both operating rooms and, therefore, the patients who were already waiting 6 months have to wait even longer, as the designated cases for the STSM are done. This is also violation of rights-based justice, and a patient's right to health care.

An alternative approach to diverting resources and destabilizing a health care system is to engage in the public health agenda to drive global surgery forward. This includes engagement with local stakeholders and collaborations with health care systems with the end goal of improving care for surgical patients.

SUMMARY

Surgical organizations can make substantial contributions to eliminating the disparity in global surgery, specifically in developing nations. The goal of eliminating disparities has ethical foundations in the principle of justice.[43] There has been debate about what constitutes universal ethical principles, and whether principles can be universally applicable. The standard, medical ethical principles described herein can help us to establish a foundation that transcends borders and cultures.

With the effort to make global surgery a worldwide initiative, it is important that as these contributions are made, we follow the ethical principles of autonomy, beneficence, nonmaleficence, and justice. We must adapt a common moral language and translate that into a common moral practice if we are to see the optimal result from efforts to eliminate the gap and increase access to high-quality surgical care. If we do not behold ethical principles and exploit the individuals we seek to help, we are likely to see unintended consequences of decreased access, unaffordable, and low-quality surgical services in low-resource settings.

Despite limitations of STSMs, including their short duration and lack of long-term collaboration and questionable sustainability, establishing a continuous long-term relationship can be key to transcending these limitations. Long-term collaborations facilitate training, education, and can help in establishing and building trust. Debas[44] states that this is the perfect time to make global surgery a worldwide initiative driven by US academic institutions, surgical organizations, and other societies, including anesthesia and nursing. Global surgery, which includes short-term work, also includes the establishment of these long-term partnerships. Academic global surgery serves the purpose of training, research, and efforts to alleviate the global disparity in ensuring access to high-quality, cost-effective surgical care in light of economic and political challenges encountered in many developing nations.[45] This can only be done with collaboration and partnerships. The same approach should be taken when we set out for STSMs, for we are in effect partnering with local surgeons to continue high-quality care delivery.

Our local surgeons and contemporaries are not inferior and are more astute than one may assume. As we leave our institutions and our respective countries, to venture to "do good" in accordance with the Hippocratic oath, it is of the utmost importance that we hold ourselves to the same standards and aim to deliver high-quality care, in abidance with the ethical principles of autonomy, beneficence and nonmaleficence, and justice. These principles, which are cross-cultural and cross borders, apply irrespective of where we are practicing.

REFERENCES

1. Shrime MG, Bickler SW, Alkire BC, et al. Global burden of surgical disease: an estimation from the provider perspective. Lancet Glob Health 2015; 3(Suppl 2):S8–9.
2. Meara JG, Leather AJ, Hagander L, et al. Global Surgery 2030: evidence and solutions for achieving health, welfare, and economic development. Lancet 2015;386(9993):569–624.
3. Bickler SN, Weiser TG, Kassebaum N, et al. Global burden of surgical conditions. In: Debas HT, Donkor P, Gawande A, et al, editors. Essential surgery: disease control priorities, third edition, vol. 1. Washington, DC: The International Bank for Reconstruction and Development/The World Bank; 2015. p. 19–40.
4. Weiser TG, Regenbogen SE, Thompson KD, et al. An estimation of the global volume of surgery: a modelling strategy based on available data. Lancet 2008;372(9633):139–44.
5. de Putter CE, van Beeck EF, Polinder S, et al. Healthcare costs and productivity costs of hand and wrist injuries by external cause: a population-based study in working-age adults in the period 2008-2012. Injury 2016;47(7):1478–82.
6. Benatar SR. Imperialism, research ethics and global health. J Med Ethics 1998;24(4):221–2.
7. Institute of Medicine Board on International Health. America's vital interest in global health: protecting our people, enhancing our economy, and advancing our international interests. Washington, DC: National Academies Press; 1997.
8. Beauchamp TL, Childress JF. Principles of biomedical ethics. USA: Oxford University Press; 2013.
9. Grimes CE, Namboya F. Ethics of global health care. Int Anesthesiol Clin 2015;53(3):90–7.
10. Gillon R. Medical ethics: four principles plus attention to scope. BMJ 1994;309(6948):184–8.
11. Association of American Medical Colleges (AAMC). Matriculating student questionnaire: 2014 all schools summary report. Washington, DC: Association of American Medical Colleges; 2014.
12. Powell AC, Casey K, Liewehr DJ, et al. Results of a national survey of surgical resident interest in international experience, electives, and volunteerism. J Am Coll Surg 2009;208(2):304–12.
13. Bale AG, Sifri ZC. Surgery resident participation in short-term humanitarian international surgical missions can supplement exposure where program case volumes are low. Am J Surg 2016;211(1):294–9.
14. Gishen K, Thaller SR. Surgical mission trips as an educational opportunity for medical students. J Craniofac Surg 2015;26(4):1095–6.
15. Dacso M, Chandra A, Friedman H. Adopting an ethical approach to global health training: the evolution of the Botswana-University of Pennsylvania partnership. Acad Med 2013;88(11):1646–50.
16. Jarman BT, Cogbill TH, Kitowski NJ. Development of an international elective in a general surgery residency. J Surg Educ 2009;66(4):222–4.
17. Campbell A, Sullivan M, Sherman R, et al. The medical mission and modern cultural competency training. J Am Coll Surg 2011;212(1):124–9.

18. Crump JA, Sugarman J. Ethics and best practice guidelines for training experiences in global health. Am J Trop Med Hyg 2010;83(6):1178–82.

19. Crump JA, Sugarman J. Ethical considerations for short-term experiences by trainees in global health. JAMA 2008;300(12):1456–8.

20. DeCamp M, Rodriguez J, Hecht S, et al. An ethics curriculum for short-term global health trainees. Global Health 2013;9:5.

21. Elobu AE, Kintu A, Galukande M, et al. Evaluating international global health collaborations: perspectives from surgery and anesthesia trainees in Uganda. Surgery 2014;155(4):585–92.

22. Abdelwahab HH, Shigidi MM, Ibrahim LS, et al. Barriers to kidney transplantation among adult Sudanese patients on maintenance hemodialysis in dialysis units in Khartoum State. Saudi J Kidney Dis Transpl 2013;24(5):1044–9.

23. Grudziak J, Snock C, Zalinga T, et al. Pre-burn malnutrition increases operative mortality in burn patients who undergo early excision and grafting in a sub-Saharan African burn unit. Burns 2018;44(3):692–9.

24. Mambou Tebou CG, Temgoua MN, Esiene A, et al. Impact of perioperative nutritional status on the outcome of abdominal surgery in a sub-Saharan Africa setting. BMC Res Notes 2017;10(1):484.

25. Hesse AA, Nouri A, Hassan HS, et al. Parasitic infestations requiring surgical interventions. Semin Pediatr Surg 2012;21(2):142–50.

26. Khurmi N, Gorlin A, Misra L. Perioperative considerations for patients with sickle cell disease: a narrative review. Can J Anaesth 2017;64(8):860–9.

27. Wall AE. Ethics in global surgery. World J Surg 2014;38(7):1574–80.

28. Shaywitz DA, Ausiello DA. Global health: a chance for Western physicians to give-and receive. Am J Med 2002;113(4):354–7.

29. Kahn C. As 'voluntourism' explodes in popularity, who's it helping most?. In: Goats and soda: stories of life in a changing world National Public Radio. Washington, DC: Podcast; 2014.

30. Maki J, Qualls M, White B, et al. Health impact assessment and short-term medical missions: a methods study to evaluate quality of care. BMC Health Serv Res 2008;8:121.

31. Dupuis CC. Humanitarian missions in the third world: a polite dissent. Plast Reconstr Surg 2004;113(1):433–5.

32. Wall A. The context of ethical problems in medical volunteer work. HEC Forum 2011;23(2):79–90.

33. Kruk ME, Gage AD, Arsenault C, et al. High-quality health systems in the Sustainable Development Goals era: time for a revolution. Lancet Glob Health 2018;6(11):e1196–252.

34. Front Matter National Academies of Sciences E, and Medicine. Crossing the global quality chasm: improving health care worldwide. Washington, DC: The National Academies Press; 2018.

35. Nepogodiev D, Martin J, Biccard B, et al. Global burden of postoperative death. Lancet 2019;393:401.

36. World Health Organization. Guidelines for health care equipment donations 2000. Geneva (Switzerland).

37. Butler M, Drum E, Evans FM, et al. Guidelines and checklists for short-term missions in global pediatric surgery: recommendations from the American Academy of Pediatrics Delivery of Surgical Care Global Health Subcommittee, American Pediatric Surgical Association Global Pediatric Surgery Committee, Society for Pediatric Anesthesia Committee on International Education and Service, and American Pediatric Surgical Nurses Association, Inc. Global Health Special Interest Group. Paediatr Anaesth 2018;28(5):392–410.

38. Sheth NP, Donegan DJ, Foran JR, et al. Global health and orthopaedic surgery—a call for international morbidity and mortality conferences. Int J Surg case Rep 2015;6c:63–7.

39. McQueen KA, Burkle FM Jr, Al-Gobory ET, et al. Maintaining baseline, corrective surgical care during asymmetrical warfare: a case study of a humanitarian mission in the safe zone of a neighboring country. Prehosp Disaster Med 2007;22(1):3–7 [discussion: 8].

40. Johnston PF, Kunac A, Gyakobo M, et al. Short-term surgical missions in resource-limited environments: Five years of early surgical outcomes. Am J Surg 2019;217(1):7–11.

41. Gil J, Rodriguez JM, Hernandez Q, et al. Do hernia operations in African international cooperation programmes provide good quality? World J Surg 2012;36(12):2795–801.

42. Farmer PE, Kim JY. Surgery and global health: a view from beyond the OR. World J Surg 2008;32(4):533–6.

43. Dwyer J. Global health and justice. Bioethics 2005;19(5–6):460–75.

44. Debas HT. The emergence and future of global surgery in the United States. JAMA Surg 2015;150(9):833–4.

45. Schecter WP. Academic global surgery: a moral imperative. JAMA Surg 2015;150(7):605–6.

Collaboration in Outreach
The Kumasi, Ghana, Model

Brittany J. Behar, MD[a], Oheneba Owusu Danso, MD[b], Boutros Farhat, MD[c],
Vincent Ativor, MD[c], Joshua Abzug, MD[d,e], Donald H. Lalonde, MD[f,*]

KEYWORDS

- Cultural competency • Global surgery • Surgical outreach • Surgery mission • WALANT
- Field sterility • Wide-awake hand surgery

KEY POINTS

- Surgeons from North America and Ghana collaborated to establish an affordable wide-awake hand surgery room with evidence-based field sterility in Kumasi, Ghana, as it is practiced in North America.
- The hand surgery organizations American Association for Surgery of the Hand and American Society for Surgery of the Hand are collaborating with Kumasi hand surgeons, therapists, and Health Volunteers Overseas to exchange knowledge through visiting surgeons, therapists, and transatlantic videoconferencing.
- Surgical outreach trips should not only provide surgical treatment to a set of in-need patients but should also aim to share knowledge and connect with surgeons and therapists at the host facility to improve access for adequate surgical care.
- Adaptability, open-mindedness, and culturally sensitive communication are all necessary to a successful global surgery trip. These skills should be introduced and practiced by volunteer groups before embarking on organized trips.

INTRODUCTION

The burden of surgical disease in low-income and middle-income countries is increasing, with an estimated unmet need of 3300 to 6400 operations per 100,000 people.[1] Barriers to access to surgical treatment include lack of facilities, equipment, and expertise in low-income and middle-income hospitals.[2] As this unmet need is increasingly recognized, physicians and caregivers from high-income countries are participating in more and more outreach trips as a way of closing the surgical burden gap. With this growing interest, global surgery overall is transforming from short-term mission trips to long-term capacity-building partnerships.[3] A shifting paradigm is moving global surgery from a vertical model of disaster response and mission work toward building systems of surgical care, with trainee development programs as an integral part of the solution to inadequate surgical care access.[4]

This article describes a collaborative effort of Ghanaian, Canadian, and American hand surgeons and therapists; Health Volunteers Overseas (HVO); the American Association for Hand Surgery (AAHS); and the American Society for Surgery of the Hand (ASSH) to establish more affordable,

Disclosures: None of the authors have any financial disclosures.
[a] Hospital of the University of Pennsylvania, 3737 Market Street, Philadelphia, PA 19104, USA; [b] Komfo Anokye Teaching Hospital, PO Box 1934, Kumasi, Ghana; [c] Komfo Anokye Teaching Hospital, PO Box 1934, Kumasi, Ghana; [d] Department of Orthopedics, University of Maryland School of Medicine, One Texas Station Court, Suite 300, Timonium, MD 21093 USA; [e] Department of Pediatrics, University of Maryland School of Medicine, One Texas Station Court, Suite 300, Timonium, MD 21093 USA; [f] Dalhousie University, 600 Main Street Suite C204, Saint John, New Brunswick E2K 1J5, Canada
* Corresponding author.
E-mail address: dlalonde@drlalonde.ca

Hand Clin 35 (2019) 429–434
https://doi.org/10.1016/j.hcl.2019.07.009
0749-0712/19/© 2019 Elsevier Inc. All rights reserved.

hand.theclinics.com

safe, evidence-based hand surgery in Kumasi, Ghana. Surgeons from North America and Ghana collaborated to establish an affordable evidence-based field sterility wide-awake hand surgery room in Kumasi Ghana, as it is practiced in North America.[5–7] The most expensive parts of hand surgery are the sedation and the full operating room sterility.[8–10] Neither is essential for most hand surgery today.[11] The American hand surgery organizations AAHS and ASSH are collaborating with Kumasi hand surgeons and therapists and HVO to share knowledge in Kumasi through visiting surgeons and transatlantic videoconferencing on a regular basis. The long-term goal is to establish the first West African Hand Surgery fellowship in Kumasi, Ghana.

THE KUMASI, GHANA, MODEL

In 2012, the AAHS president-elect Dr Don Lalonde, in collaboration with HVO, visited Kumasi, Ghana, with the hope of establishing a reverse fellowship in hand surgery. A normal fellowship usually involves taking an international fellow to an established hand surgery center in North America or Europe. A reverse fellowship involves taking the teachers to the residents and fellows in the country where there is no established fellowship training. This concept brings knowledge to the home environment where locally trained surgeons and therapists are more likely to stay home and help people who lack access to care.

TRANS-ATLANTIC WEBINAR SERIES WITH AMERICAN ASSOCIATION FOR SURGERY OF THE HAND

The AAHS and Josh Abzug (United States) have worked with Oheneba Owusu Danso, Boutros Farhat, and Vincent Ativor of Kumasi to create a series of weekly Webinars in hand surgery and therapy that have been running successfully for 4 years. These Webinars cover the full range of hand surgery and hand therapy. They are coordinated from Baltimore and Boston and transmitted to Kumasi, Ghana, weekly, with the exception of the summer.

The AAHS formally partnered with the Komfo Anokye Teaching Hospital in Kumasi, Ghana, in 2015 to attempt to provide formal education to the attending physicians, hand surgery fellows, residents, medical students, and therapists. This relationship was initially developed based on the connection Dr Lalonde had developed following medical mission trips to this hospital. The concept was to provide a weekly conference for the care providers in Kumasi using a customary North American approach. For this to occur, a stable Internet connection would be necessary, as well as live streaming capabilities in Kumasi. The first step in assessing this was procurement of a program that would provide the opportunity to share PowerPoint slides, as well as provide a live streaming feed to another site. Essentially, a Webinar would be given on a weekly basis to the care providers in Kumasi that would enable real-time feedback to permit questions to be asked and answered, as well as discussion of any upcoming challenging cases.

Following the procurement of the appropriate software and the establishment of a time and location to give the weekly lecture series, the Internet connection was assessed and found to be suitable. The next step was the creation of an academic schedule and then obtaining the appropriate speakers. To accomplish this task, the AAHS education committee developed a curriculum for the hand surgery providers in Kumasi, analogous to a hand surgery fellowship or resident curriculum in North America, beginning with anatomy and then getting into more complex hand surgery topics. After the curriculum was developed, a survey was sent out to the membership of the AAHS to permit members to sign up for 1 to 2 lectures during the year. Within a few weeks, more than 40 members had agreed to give the approximately 50 lectures during the year. The program was now set to begin providing typical North American weekly educational conferences in an underdeveloped part of Africa.

The first several lectures were fraught with numerous issues that led to much frustration. There were times that the AAHS member and assisting staff were logged in but the colleagues in Kumasi were not, as well as times that there were Internet connection issues. Additionally, there were several weeks of holidays and funerals in Kumasi that the AAHS staff and speakers were unaware of, leading to several weeks of having a North American surgeon volunteer taking an hour out of their day after preparing a lecture and then having no one to lecture to. Occasionally, the lectures were able to be rescheduled but more often than not the lecture was just canceled. At the end of the first year, only approximately 50% of the lectures were given. However, the appreciation and acknowledgment of the colleagues in Kumasi led to the desire to continue on.

In 2016, Dr Lalonde visited Kumasi and discussed the lecture cycle with colleagues in Kumasi. Internet issues and scheduling conflicts were resolved. The AAHS and Kumasi leaders had worked out a better time and location that would be more reliable. Additionally, the AAHS staff were made aware of the various holidays in Kumasi and were able to create a schedule around them. Therefore, the second year ran much more smoothly. Colleagues in Kumasi were more engaged and able to attend many more lectures. However, approximately 20% of the lectures still had various issues, including no attendance, difficulty connecting via the Internet, and so forth.

Fortunately, the mission of the AAHS is "Working together to advance global hand care and education." As such, the collaborators have persisted and are currently beginning the fourth year of weekly lectures provided by AAHS members to Kumasi, Ghana. Over the last year, more than 90% of the scheduled lectures have been given without any issues. The attending physicians, trainees, and therapists in Kumasi are truly grateful for the education they are receiving at no cost and for the ability to interact with North American colleagues. Relationships have grown and additional sites will be added to continue to advance global hand care and education.

HAND THERAPY DEVELOPMENT IN KUMASI

Since 2014, more than a dozen hand therapists from Canada and the United States have spent at least a week in Kumasi to help begin hand therapy. Many have received funding from the AAHS. These include Gayle Severance, Heather Wood, Adam Creiling, Brian Wilkerson, Paul Bonzani, Rajani Sharma, Lisa Flewelling, Catherine Sullivan, Cynthia Cooper, Jenna Millman, Courtney Middleton, and Kelly Godwin. With their efforts, Robert Sowa has become the first dedicated hand therapist in Kumasi. He now attends hand surgery clinics with the hand surgeons in Kumasi to coordinate care of complex hand-injured patients.

SURGEONS, FELLOWS, AND PLASTIC-ORTHOPEDIC RESIDENTS WHO VISIT KUMASI FOR KNOWLEDGE EXCHANGE

Since 2014, HVO, AAHS, and ASSH have contributed a steady stream of hand surgeons, fellows, and plastic-orthopedic residents who visit Kumasi for knowledge exchange. They are dedicated to hand surgery. They spent time lecturing, operating with, and learning from the general surgery, plastic surgery, and orthopedic surgery residents and surgeons, as well as hand therapists, in Kumasi, on the care of the hand.

ESTABLISHMENT OF FIELD STERILITY

Evidence-based field sterility has been gradually replacing main operating room sterility for much of hand surgery in Canada for 40 years, with no increase in complications but a significant decrease in expense and garbage production.[12] Many surgeons in many countries have begun to move this way.[13,14]

Dr Lalonde returned to Kumasi in 2016 and 2017 to help establish wide-awake hand surgery with field sterility outside the main operating room, as it is practiced in Canada. Before that, the main operating room with obligatory full sterility and sedation were the only way to provide hand surgery. This was not financially attainable by most of the population. Discussions were held with all the surgical groups and the hospital administration in 2016 to consider adopting the North American model in which much simple hand surgery and trauma is being moved out of the main operating room to much less expensive minor procedure rooms with a wide-awake, local anesthesia, no tourniquet (WALANT) approach. The hospital administration agreed to this concept after reviewing presentations of evidence-based sterility and the North American experience.

In February of 2017, a previous burn unit room just outside of the main operating room at KATH was converted to a wide-awake hand surgery room and the first cases were performed. Since then, that room has been very busy with, not only hand surgery, but also other cases performed under local anesthesia. In the first year of its existence, more than 360 surgeries were performed in that room at a much lower cost for local patients who can now afford hand reconstruction after injuries.

ESTABLISHMENT OF A WEST AFRICAN HAND SURGERY FELLOWSHIP PROGRAM

Dr Brad Rockwell (University of Utah, Salt Lake City, Utah) is working in collaboration with the Dr Lalonde, the AAHS, the ASSH, Dr Oheneba Owusu-Danso, Dr Paa Ekow Hoyte-Williams, Dr Boutros Farhat, and Dr Pius Agbenorku of the Ghana College of Physicians and Surgeons to establish the first hand surgery fellowship site in Northwest Africa in Kumasi, Ghana. The model works on the reverse fellowship type format in which North Americans collaborate with Ghanaians to make this happen in Ghana.

DISCUSSION

Hand surgery does not have to be expensive. The advent of evidence-based sterility and wide-awake hand surgery has greatly reduced the cost of hand surgery and the need for sedation. This article discusses how North American hand surgeons have collaborated with hand surgeons from Ghana to help establish new educational models that use the Internet and a structured visiting surgeon and therapist program to improve hand care and accessibility to patients in Ghana using these new advances. Programs of this kind must be established with cultural sensitivity and competency.

Cultural competency is defined as an elevated level of knowledge of and appropriate response to varying cultures that allows health care workers to interact with patients from various cultural backgrounds.[15] This skill provides health care workers with an approach for being receptive, empathetic, and compassionate to a variety of ideas, customs, and lifestyles of the patients they are treating.[16] Tervalon and Murray-Garcia[17] note that a better implementation of this in clinical practice is a commitment and an active engagement in a lifelong process that physicians embark on with their patients rather than a discrete endpoint. Curriculums designed to focus on cultural competence aim to increase students' awareness of their own cultural backgrounds and other cultures via self-reflection, cultural vignettes, and shared narratives.[18]

Four specific elements contribute to cultural competency: (1) culturally appropriate communication, (2) situational and self-awareness, (3) adaptability, and (4) knowledge about core cultural issues.[19] Cultural norms may dictate what behavior is acceptable; for example, what questions are appropriate to ask during a patient history and examination, what attire is worn (or not) in the operating suite, and what level of supervision is acceptable for trainees during surgery. Appropriate communication can dictate a patient's comfort level with the surgery. For instance, several investigators showed that 9% to 33% of patients in foreign countries are afraid of surgery.[2] However, in 1 study, changing the description for eye surgery to washing of cataract increased patients' willingness to have a procedure.[20] Patients may also have specific cultural beliefs surrounding a specific surgical condition or feel that traditional healers are better equipped to treat them. For example, a belief that blindness from cataracts is God's will or is due to witchcraft and thus incurable will prevent patients from seeking surgical treatment.[21] Students and physicians may anticipate differences in clothing and food but may not anticipate the major differences in cultural values in medical treatment expressed at the local hospitals compared with those at their home institution.[22] It is critical to prepare for any outreach trip by focusing on honing these skills and anticipating the unanticipated.

Global health trips teach visiting physicians to understand resource allocation and system-based medicine, especially in regions that lack adequate access to surgical care. Physicians must have several operative options in anticipation of lack of access to equipment normally available at home institutions. Treating a surgical problem with little to no equipment is critical to a successful trip. It must be highlighted though that global surgery trips can evolve into medical tourism easily. Medical tourism is defined as "participation in an international clinical health experience in a resource-poor destination by a trainee from a high-income country where the net gain favors the trainee participant and insufficient consideration is given to the needs...of the host country."[23] Establishing clear-cut goals before departure, adequately educating the volunteering medical team, and anticipating the needs of the host country can help avoid this imbalanced experience. Understanding that certain resources are sometimes unavailable, such as fluoroscopy, a surgical microscope, or a specific necessary suture, can temper patient and hospital expectations. Operative management plans shared with the host surgical team are more likely to be implemented after the visiting team when less complex solutions are offered.[24]

Surgeons must not only travel and operate with relevant skills and knowledge but also with ethical and legal expectations of standard practices.[25] It is critical that surgeons try to uphold their standard of ethical and moral treatment of their foreign patients, even if unethical treatment is accepted otherwise. The best surgical treatment options, considering all resources available, should always be offered, even if it is more difficult or complex. Although malpractice is rare and unlikely, the volunteer physician should uphold his or her standards despite this in all operative endeavors they pursue.

SUMMARY

Global surgical outreach trips are growing in popularity. The primary goal of these trips is shifting from short-term surgical treatment of a select group, to more sustainable surgical interventions, including setting up of uncomplicated facilities, focusing on resident and health care worker education, and establishing long-term working relationships between lower income hospitals and high-income facilities. These goals are contingent on mutual respect among care takers, as well as open-mindedness toward host country's teaching styles, trainee expectations, patients' cultural understanding of their diseases, and adaptability to acute situations, including lack of necessary instruments and supplies.

Without these skill sets, physicians are unable to become culturally competent and fulfill their goals during surgical mission work. Volunteers should receive education and training before global outreach trips focusing on how to be adaptable and open-minded, and how to use culturally appropriate communication. Without these skills, volunteers may become frustrated or feel unfilled with their experience and avoid additional outreach projects. A little preparation and training can make volunteer experiences even more fulfilling and promote more long-lasting relationships between the host medical team and the visiting medical team.

REFERENCES

1. Rose J, Weiser TG, Hider P, et al. Estimated need for surgery worldwide based on prevalence of diseases: implications for public health planning of surgical services. Lancet Glob Health 2015;3(Suppl 2): S13–20.
2. Grimes CE, Bowman KG, Dodgion CM, et al. Systematic review of barriers to surgical care in low-income and middle-income countries. World J Surg 2011;35:941–50.
3. Chao TE, Riesel JN, Anderson GA, et al. Building a global surgery initiative through evaluation, collaboration, and training: the Massachusetts General Hospital Experience. J Surg Educ 2015; 72(4):e21–8.
4. Farmer P, Meara JG. Commentary: The agenda for academic excellence in "global" surgery. Surgery 2013;153:321–2.
5. Alam M, Ibrahim O, Nodzenski M, et al. Adverse events associated with Mohs micrographic surgery: multicenter prospective cohort study of 20,821 cases at 23 centers. JAMA Dermatol 2013;149: 1378.
6. Leblanc MR, Lalonde DH, Thoma A, et al. Is main operating room sterility really necessary in carpal tunnel surgery? A multicenter prospective study of minor procedure room field sterility surgery. Hand (N Y) 2011;6:60.
7. Garon MT, Massey P, Chen A1, et al. Cost and complications of percutaneous fixation of hand fractures in a procedure room versus the operating room. Hand (N Y) 2018;13(4):428–34.
8. Leblanc MR, Lalonde J, Lalonde DH. A detailed cost and efficiency analysis of performing carpal tunnel surgery in the main operating room versus the ambulatory setting in Canada. Hand (N Y) 2007;2:173.
9. Sieber D, Lacey A, Fletcher J, et al. Cost savings using minimal draping for routine hand procedures. Minn Med 2014;97:49.
10. Bismil MS, Bismil QM, Harding D, et al. Transition to total one-stop wide-awake hand surgery service-audit: a retrospective review. JRSM Short Rep 2012;3:23.
11. Lalonde DH. Conceptual origins, current practice and views of wide awake hand surgery. J Hand Surg Eur Vol 2017;42(9):886–95.
12. Lalonde DH. Field sterility for simple cases makes sense. In: Lalonde DH, editor. Wide awake hand surgery. New York: Thieme; 2016. p. 69–73.
13. Chatterjee A, McCarthy JE, Montagne SA, et al. A cost, profit, and efficiency analysis of performing carpal tunnel surgery in the operating room versus the clinic setting in the United States. Ann Plast Surg 2011;66:245.
14. Dua K, Blevins CJ, O'Hara NN, et al. The safety and benefits of the semisterile technique for closed reduction and percutaneous pinning of pediatric upper extremity fractures. Hand (N Y) 2018. [Epub ahead of print].
15. Flores G. Culture and the patient-physician relationship: achieving cultural competency in health care. J Pediatr 2000;136:14–23.
16. Butler PD, Swift M, Kothari S, et al. Integrating cultural competency and humility training into clinical clerkships: surgery as a model. J Surg Educ 2011; 68:222–30.
17. Tervalon M, Murray-Garcia J. Cultural humility versus cultural competence: a critical distinction in defining physician training outcomes in multicultural education. J Health Care Poor Underserved 1998;9(2): 117–25.
18. Kutob RM, Bormanis J, Crago M, et al. Cultural competence education for practicing physicians: lessons in cultural humility, nonjudgmental behaviors and health beliefs elicitation. J Contin Educ Health Prof 2013;33(3):164–73.
19. Teal CR, Street RL. Critical elements of culturally competent communication in the medical encounter: a review and model. Soc Sci Med 2009;68:533–43.
20. Ojabo CO, Alao O. Cataract surgery: limitations and barriers in Makurdi, Benue State. Niger J Med 2009; 18:250–5.
21. Bronsard A, Geneau R, Shirima S, et al. Why are children brought late for cataracts surgery? Qualitative findings from Tanzania. Ophthalmic Epidemiol 2008;14:383–8.

22. Mutabdzic D, Azzie G. Uncovering the hidden curriculum of global health electives. Ann Surg 2016; 263(5):853–4.

23. Petrosoniak A, McCarthy A, Varpio L. International health electives: thematic results of student and professional interviews. Med Educ 2010;44:683–9.

24. Kozin SH. Surgeons beyond borders: techniques revived in an underserved area. Tech Hand Upper Extrem Surg 2007;11(3):209–13.

25. Monsudi KF, Oladel TO, Naisr AA, et al. Medical ethics in sub-Saharan Africa: closing the gaps. Afr Health Sc 2015;15(2):673–81.

International Partnerships for Hand Surgery Education

George S.M. Dyer, MD

KEYWORDS

- Global surgery • International orthopedics • Surgical education • Volunteer

KEY POINTS

- Surgical care is a major unmet need in global health.
- Hand surgery is an important component of that need.
- Carefully planned, long-term partnerships can build surgical capacity in developing countries.
- Participating in such partnerships is well within the capacity of many practicing hand surgeons in North America.

Nurturing worldwide capacity to perform surgery of the hand and upper extremity has unique potential to improve health in low-income and middle-income countries. Even aside from the management of acute injuries to the hand, many upper extremity–trained surgeons possess other skills critical to treating a range of skeletal conditions in a low-resource environment. Examples include:

- Soft tissue management, such as flaps, grafts, and other coverage techniques
- Familiarity with nerve injury and repair
- Management of chronic injury to small joints, such as contracture, tendon ruptures, lacerations, and adhesions
- Congenital and developmental conditions of the hand or upper extremity, such as congenital difference, brachial plexus birth palsy, and injuries sustained while still growing

The worldwide burden of musculoskeletal injury is immense, and it can be reduced by the thoughtful volunteer efforts of individual surgeons. Mission-style visits to developing countries are a mainstay of volunteer engagement and these are cost-effective and useful. Even better, and increasing in number, are sustained partnerships to teach local surgeons and to build surgical capacity.

BACKGROUND

The potential benefit of this work is measured by the scope of untreated injury and global unmet need for surgery. Consider that traumatic injuries kill more people worldwide than human immunodeficiency virus/acquired immunodeficiency syndrome, malaria, and tuberculosis combined, and almost all of these patients with trauma are poor and young.[1–6] For every 1 death caused by trauma, many more survive with disability, contributing to a vicious cycle of poverty for individuals and communities[7,8] Many of those injuries involve the upper extremity. Deprived of a functioning hand, options for productive work are particularly diminished in low-resource economies.

This burden becomes more visible during humanitarian crises. Humanitarian crises directly affected 144 million people worldwide in 2012.[9] To this grim tally, add injuries deliberately inflicted during armed conflict, genocide, and civil war.[10,11]

Funding has included the ASSH and AAOS (directly for HAAOT), the FOT (both for the missions mentioned and for HAAOT), and ASSH for Touching Hands Project.
Department of Orthopaedic Surgery, Brigham and Women's Hospital, 75 Francis Street, Boston, MA 02115, USA
E-mail address: gdyer@mgh.harvard.edu

Hand Clin 35 (2019) 435–440
https://doi.org/10.1016/j.hcl.2019.07.007

For example, during the genocidal Rwandan civil conflict, ritualistic maiming of the hands was used repeatedly as a terror tactic.

In straightforward economic cost, the burden is tremendous. A 2015 modeling study suggested that injuries could result in $7.9 trillion in cumulative gross domestic product losses caused by decreased economic productivity between 2015 and 2030, with losses in low-income and middle-income countries often 50% greater than in high-income countries (HICs).[12]

A BLUEPRINT FOR HELPING

A comprehensive solution would require national-level policy steps to reduce injury and mortality. The rudimentary resources for safe surgery include stable electric power, clean water, and the capacity to maintain sterility. Beyond this, competent anesthesia and nursing services are essential. Fixing all of this is beyond the scope or capacity of individual surgeons, but improving access to quality surgical care is an important step.[13]

Even incremental improvements in basic orthopedic care lead to proven benefits. For example, open fractures can be successfully treated using the same standardized protocols developed in HICs of primary external fixation, sequential debridements, and early use of local muscle or fasciocutaneous flaps for soft tissue coverage. The coverage component is a particular challenge in low-resource settings, where a disproportionate number of injuries are open and require coverage. Upper extremity surgeons, trained in soft tissue management techniques, offer particularly valuable expertise.[14]

Orthopedic mission trips, both elective and for disaster relief, seem to be safe[15,16] and cost-effective compared with other important global health interventions,[17,18] especially for hand or upper extremity–focused missions.[19]

However, focusing just on doing surgery can be a trap, and potentially causes harm. If a visiting team of surgeons performs a series of complex operations during a brief mission visit, who follows those patients afterward, or treats the inevitable complications? A moral hazard is that well-meaning visiting surgeons can perpetuate a cycle of dependency in the places they are trying to assist.[20]

Consider the following:

- Visiting surgeons displace local staff, both immediately during their visit and also afterward.
- Donated expertise and equipment, typically offered for free during the mission, compete unfairly with local surgeons. How can they possibly compete with visiting experts, perhaps world-famous experts, who charge zero?
- Dependence on external assistance reduces access in the long term, as patients seek out providers of free care, whereas local surgeons leave for areas without competitors.[21]

The most beneficial and successful surgical missions are integrated with the local care delivery system. They are explicitly designed to develop local surgical capacity and effectively put themselves out of business over time.[22]

There are many examples of programs engineered for constructive engagement and they each have most or all of the following characteristics:

1. Focused on education
   a. Education is the most valuable and durable gift a mission can provide, helping host surgeons learn new techniques and teach others, disseminating knowledge and best practices even further.[23]
2. Partnership is sustained over time
   a. This characteristic also supports good medical care. Local partners are essential to complete the care of patients after visiting surgeons have returned home.[24]
3. Two-way exchange of ideas and expertise
4. Partnership includes more than just surgeons and other doctors

SOME ILLUSTRATIVE EXAMPLES

Here are a few examples of partnerships that have been successful over time in one nearby country, Haiti. It is important to stress that these are not the only examples of good initiatives there. It would be impossible to offer a comprehensive list of all the great projects taking place even in that single country; other examples or other countries could have been chosen just as well, and no insult is intended. However, these are selected examples principles that may be generalized into a useful template.

TOUCHING HANDS PROJECT

Founded in 2013 by then president of the American Society for Surgery of the Hand, Dr Scott Kozin, the pilot mission of the Touching Hands Project was to Haiti in July 2014. That pilot mission included all of the elements that have come to characterize the Touching Hands Project.

It included 3 experienced orthopedic hand surgeons, and 1 fellow. The trip was only a week long, but more than 2 months of careful planning

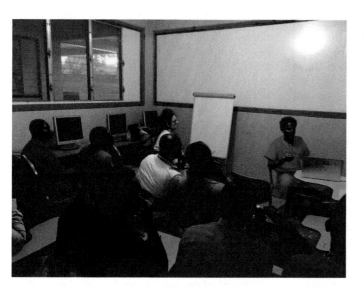

Fig. 1. Teaching during a Touching Hand Project visit to Haiti.

beforehand went into it. The recipient site, Adventist Hospital near Port-au-Prince in Haiti, had a long history of productive partnership with visiting foreign surgeons. The Haitian chief of orthopedic surgery of the hospital, Dr Francel Alexis, is one of a handful of fellowship-trained pediatric orthopedic surgeons in the country. Dr Alexis arranged for patients with the most complex surgical needs to travel to Port-au-Prince for surgical consultation and operation during the team's visit.

The team was not limited to surgeons. There were also experienced anesthesiologists capable of performing regional anesthesia so that upper limb surgery could be performed in many cases without the need of general anesthesia. Perioperative nurses were part of the team, and they partnered with nurses from the host facility throughout the visit.

Perhaps most important, the team included experienced occupational therapists, whose own professional organization had a long-term parallel engagement in the same area. This arrangement permitted immediate on-site patient education for postoperative exercises, and it also guaranteed built-in follow-up of the most complex cases in 6 months and then a year, with treating therapists well versed in the protocols.

That basic formula has been repeated in Haiti annually, with trips of slightly varying configurations. Dr Jeffrey Gelfand has led an annual series of visits to the same hospital, which permits follow-up for individual patients. More importantly, consistent partnership has deepened ties not only between the surgeons but also with the nurses and other professionals involved over time. Education has been, from the start, a central feature of the

visits. Although the surgery has all taken place in 1 hospital, surgical trainees from throughout the region of the Haitian capital travel to that hospital during the week of the mission in order to scrub cases and discuss them. The week features a formal lecture series with talks given in English and, when possible, in French by visiting faculty (**Fig. 1**).

Not limited to Haiti, the Touching Hands Project has expanded to include more than 40 trips to 13 different countries, including several domestic missions to treat the underserved within the United States.

FOUNDATION FOR ORTHOPEDIC TRAUMA

The Foundation for Orthopedic Trauma (FOT) is an academic organization dedicated to the improvement of trauma care by direct education of trainees and practicing surgeons, and by sponsoring research. It has a well-planned humanitarian outreach component, and since the Haitian earthquake of 2010, that outreach has focused particularly on Haiti. Although FOT is a general orthopedic trauma organization, its Haiti mission has been led by Dr Melvin Rosenwasser, a hand surgeon and the director of Columbia University's hand fellowship. Over 8 years, the mission has taken on something of an upper extremity focus. The FOT involvement has followed a similar pattern to the Touching Hands Project. Visiting teams are not too large, but they include other specialties other than surgeons. Hand therapists, anesthesiologists, and perioperative care nurses; each team formed partnerships with their local counterparts. Education is an explicit focus, and surgical trainees from around the region come to the hospital during its mission week, and for afternoon and evening lectures as well.

Not coincidentally, the FOT missions have settled on the same hospital partner as the Touching Hands Project in Haiti; this is not because the Adventist Hospital is the only good place for long-term partnership. Everyone involved in both teams is careful to avoid the appearance of playing favorites. By universal agreement, the facilities of the Adventist Hospital have been opened to trainees from throughout the region during these visits. However, choosing a good partner hospital and sticking with it has had definite benefits that are worth considering. The technical and nursing staff, from sterile processing to janitorial services and supply, have become more expert over the years. One young man at the hospital, originally hired as a cleaner, became interested in the more technical aspects of surgical care and, inspired by the ongoing partnership, pursued training as a surgical technologist. A single visit might not have inspired him, but sustained partnership did.

Consistent partnership also provides continuity between different visitor groups and cooperation between them. They can hand off particularly complex, multistage cases and follow up on each other's work.

HAITIAN ANNUAL CONFERENCE ON ORTHOPEDIC TRAUMATOLOGY

The Assemblée Annuelle Haitienne de Traumatologie Orthopedique (Haitian Annual Conference on Orthopedic Traumatology [HAAOT]) is an international orthopedic conference, conducted each spring in Haiti in French and English. It brings together most of Haiti's practicing orthopedic surgeons, trainees from Haiti's 3 residency training programs, and a visiting faculty from overseas. This conference is not a clinical visit, but HAAOT has become an unexpected cornerstone of one program to support and nurture development of orthopedic surgery in that country (**Fig. 2**).[25]

The conference was first organized in 2012 and launched in 2013. Conducted annually in April or May, the meeting brings together Haitian orthopedic residents and attending surgeons from across the island as well as an international faculty. Half the speakers are Haitian. The topics are chosen each year by asking the Haitian participants what they want to learn. Central themes have included management of open fracture, treatment of delayed or neglected injury, osteomyelitis, and national disaster preparedness. Before the initiation of this conference there were few venues for formal continuing medical education for orthopedic surgeons in Haiti, and no occasion when all the orthopedic practitioners and trainees in the country were invited to gather together.

The conference has been successful both at learning what Haitian participants perceive as their own knowledge gaps and also at ensuring those gaps are bridged. An anonymous electronic audience response system automates identification of learning priorities for each year.[26] This polling revealed that upper extremity themes are consistently among the most requested: soft tissue coverage for open wounds, injury to the hand, and articular injury around the elbow. The same system allows participants to answer quizzes

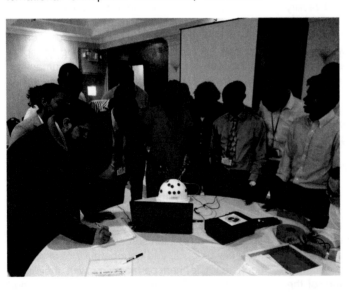

Fig. 2. Arthroscopy training at HAAOT.

confidentially and without fear of embarrassment, so understanding and retention can be assessed in real time. Response rates have consistently been 75% to 85%, and have shown immediate[27] and sustained learning.[28]

The meeting has grown rapidly in attendance, scope, and sophistication over 5 years, and now welcomes nearly100 participants, with an increasing percentage of Haitian presentations. More important than the raw number in attendance, the HAAOT has been especially effective in building participation among surgeons who would otherwise not interact.

The greatest success of HAAOT has been its contribution to creating a sense of a Haitian orthopedic community, particularly within the vibrant young generation of current Haitian orthopedic residents. By gathering them together year after year on a predictable schedule, the conference has provided a forum for them to share experiences, to benefit from each other's experience managing common and complex problems they all face, to discuss their complications honestly, and to work toward a rigorous, multicenter approach to improving care. Participants have shown objective, durable improvements in their understanding of orthopedic disorders and surgical management.[29]

SUMMARY

Through carefully planned engagement, hand and upper extremity surgeons can contribute meaningfully to improving health in low-resource countries. The 3 programs described here exemplify a few of the features that make a success of initiatives like this: centered on education, long-term partnership, and focus on building capacity beyond just surgeons. Anesthesia, nursing, sterile processing, and biomedical engineering are also important partners. The need is evident, and it is gratifying to see how many surgeons have answered the call to help.

REFERENCES

1. Agarwal-Harding KJ, von Keudell A, Zirkle LG, et al. Understanding and addressing the global need for orthopaedic trauma care. J Bone Joint Surg Am 2016;98:1844–53.
2. Koplan JP, Bond TC, Merson MH, et al. Towards a common definition of global health. Lancet 2009; 373:1993–5.
3. Farmer PE, Kim JY. Surgery and global health: a view from beyond the OR. World J Surg 2008;32: 533–6.
4. Lozano R, Naghavi M, Foreman K, et al. Global and regional mortality from 235 causes of death for 20 age groups in 1990 and 2010: a systematic analysis for the Global Burden of Disease Study 2010. Lancet 2012;380:2095–128.
5. Debas HT, Gosselin R, McCord C, et al. Surgery. In: Jamison DT, Breman JG, et al, editors. Disease control priorities in developing countries. 2006. Washington, DC.
6. Patton GC, Coffey C, Sawyer SM, et al. Global patterns of mortality in young people: a systematic analysis of population health data. Lancet 2009;374: 881–92.
7. Gosselin RA, Spiegel DA, Coughlin R, et al. Injuries: the neglected burden in developing countries. Bull World Health Organ 2009;87. 246–246a.
8. Vos T, Flaxman AD, Naghavi M, et al. Years lived with disability (YLDs) for 1160 sequelae of 289 diseases and injuries 1990-2010: a systematic analysis for the Global Burden of Disease Study 2010. Lancet 2012; 380:2163–96.
9. Smith J, Roberts B, Knight A, et al. A systematic literature review of the quality of evidence for injury and rehabilitation interventions in humanitarian crises. Int J Public Health 2015;60:865–72.
10. Leaning J, Guha-Sapir D. Natural disasters, armed conflict, and public health. N Engl J Med 2013; 369:1836–42.
11. Centers for Disease Control and Prevention (CDC). Post-earthquake injuries treated at a field hospital — Haiti, 2010. MMWR Morb Mortal Wkly Rep 2011;59:1673–7.
12. Alkire BC, Shrime MG, Dare AJ, et al. Global economic consequences of selected surgical diseases: a modelling study. Lancet Glob Health 2015;3(Suppl 2):S21–7.
13. Mock C, Cherian MN. The global burden of musculoskeletal injuries: challenges and solutions. Clin Orthop Relat Res 2008;466:2306–16.
14. Bach O, Hope MJ, Chaheka CV, et al. Disability can be avoided after open fractures in Africa-results from Malawi. Injury 2004;35:846–51.
15. Usoro AO, Bhashyam A, Mohamadi A, et al. Clinical outcomes and complications of the surgical implant generation network (SIGN) intramedullary nail: a systematic review and meta-analysis. J Orthop Trauma 2019;33:42–8.
16. Young S, Lie SA, Hallan G, et al. Low infection rates after 34,361 intramedullary nail operations in 55 low- and middle-income countries: validation of the Surgical Implant Generation Network (SIGN) online surgical database. Acta Orthop 2011;82: 737–43.
17. Gosselin RA, Gialamas G, Atkin DM. Comparing the cost-effectiveness of short orthopedic missions in elective and relief situations in developing countries. World J Surg 2011;35:951–5.

18. Chen AT, Pedtke A, Kobs JK, et al. Volunteer orthopedic surgical trips in Nicaragua: a cost-effectiveness evaluation. World J Surg 2012;36:2802–8.

19. Tadisina KK, Chopra K, Tangredi J, et al. Helping hands: a cost-effectiveness study of a humanitarian hand surgery mission. Plast Surg Int 2014;2014: 921625.

20. Welling DR, Ryan JM, Burris DG, et al. Seven sins of humanitarian medicine. World J Surg 2010;34: 466–70.

21. Green T, Green H, Scandlyn J, et al. Perceptions of short-term medical volunteer work: a qualitative study in Guatemala. Global Health 2009;5:4.

22. Patel PB, Hoyler M, Maine R, et al. An opportunity for diagonal development in global surgery: cleft lip and palate care in resource-limited settings. Plast Surg Int 2012;2012:892437.

23. Carey JN, Caldwell AM, Coughlin RR, et al. Building Orthopaedic Trauma Capacity: IGOT International SMART Course. J Orthop Trauma 2015;29(Suppl 10):S17–9.

24. Wall LL, Arrowsmith SD, Lassey AT, et al. Humanitarian ventures or 'fistula tourism?': the ethical perils of pelvic surgery in the developing world. Int Urogynecol J Pelvic Floor Dysfunct 2006;17:559–62.

25. Dyer GSM. Haitian annual conference on orthopaedic traumatology: building surgical capacity through academic collaboration. J Orthop Trauma 2018; 32(Suppl 7):S16–7.

26. Qudsi RA, Roberts HJ, Bhashyam AR, et al. A self-reported needs assessment survey of pediatric orthopaedic education in haiti. J Surg Educ 2018;75: 140–6.

27. Fils J, Bhashyam AR, Pierre JB, et al. Short-term performance improvement of a continuing medical education program in a low-income country. World J Surg 2015;39:2407–12.

28. Bhashyam AR, Fils J, Lowell J, et al. A novel approach for needs assessment to build global orthopedic surgical capacity in a low-income country. J Surg Educ 2015;72:e2–8.

29. Bhashyam AR, Logan C, Roberts HJ, et al. A randomized controlled pilot study of educational techniques in teaching basic arthroscopic skills in a low-income country. Arch Bone Jt Surg 2017;5: 82–8.

Hand Surgery in Underserved Populations in the United States

The Author's Experience with the Navajo at the Gallup and Chinle Indian Health Service Hospitals

Marco Rizzo, MD

KEYWORDS

- Hand surgery • Indian health service • Navajo

KEY POINTS

- Sharing an experience of hand surgery domestic outreach, specifically my experience with the Navajo People.
- The need and scope of problem of access to medical care at the Indian reservation is significant.
- Volunteerism and outreach are truly gratifying experiences, satisfying that desire to help in its purest form.

INTRODUCTION

Domestic health care volunteerism has a long history in the United States. Whether it occurs on a local level or more broadly in pockets of the population, the spirit of helping those who have less/no means is closely intertwined to our noble profession. I was first exposed to volunteerism in medical school at Temple University. In the late 1800s, Temple was founded as a charity hospital and has a long history of being linked to the Shriner's Hospital of Philadelphia, which offers free health care to its patients. Outreach was also an important part of my orthopedic residency at Duke University. Drs Lenox Baker and Leonard Goldner had established outreach clinics to offer orthopedic care to underserved areas in eastern rural North Carolina. Residents accompanied faculty to clinics to such places as Goldsboro, Wilson, Lumberton, and Pinehurst. These clinics offered access for patients and educational opportunities for trainees. Outreach clinics like these exist throughout the country and remain wonderful opportunities for us to help people in need.

It is often hard to predict the profound impact of seemly, at the time, innocuous events on our journeys through our careers and life. As a young hand surgeon, I had an opportunity to travel to the Navajo Nation through an American Association of Hand Surgery sponsored lecture series that included a hand surgeon and hand therapists. Paul Brach (a certified hand therapist from Pittsburgh) and I traveled to Shiprock, New Mexico and Tuba City, Arizona and provided lectures to emergency department and primary care physicians about hand-related conditions, injuries, and their care. Although we were there only 2 days, I quickly learned about the difficulties and challenges facing these providers and their patients regarding access to hand surgery and hand

Disclosure Statement: The author has no relevant conflicts related to the content of this article.
Department of Orthopedic Surgery, Division of Hand Surgery, Mayo Clinic, 200 First Street Southwest, Rochester, MN 55905, USA
E-mail address: Rizzo.marco@mayo.edu

Hand Clin 35 (2019) 441–448
https://doi.org/10.1016/j.hcl.2019.07.014

therapy care. It is hard to believe that I am now approaching 15 years since that trip and that I have been going to the reservation ever since.

THE NAVAJO NATION

The Navajo Nation is the largest Indian reservation in the country. Geographically, it is larger than the state of West Virginia. The Navajo population is estimated to be 360,000 individuals, of which approximately half live on the reservation. It encompasses a postage stamp portion of northeastern Arizona north of interstate 40, the southeastern edge of Utah, and northwestern corner of New Mexico (also generally north of interstate 40). Within the Arizona portion of the Navajo Nation lies the Hopi Reservation. The reservation is adjacent to some of the most spectacular scenery and beloved national parks in the United States including: the Grand Canyon (west), the Grand Escalante Staircase National Park (north), Petrified Forest National Park (south), and Chaco National Monument (east).

This area of land is high desert with wide open vistas, mesas, and smaller canyons. The Navajo Nation itself also includes some of the most dramatic landscape in North America including: Monument Valley, the Painted Desert, Canyon De Chelley National Monument (**Fig. 1**), and Shiprock Peak. The vistas are dramatic and the night sky is incredible to behold.

Many inhabitants of the Navajo raise sheep (**Fig. 2**) and goats and the resulting wool is sold or processed to create arts, rugs, and blankets. Although not as common nowadays, in the mid to latter part of the twentieth century, their economy was fueled by mining of coal and uranium.

Tourism is currently an important part of their economy, with approximately 3 million tourists annually.

Like many reservations throughout North America, the poverty is palpable. Approximately 50% of Navajo have no electricity or running water. Many have no telephones and communication is via mail, which they check once per week or in longer intervals at their local Post Office Boxes. According to DiscoverNavajo.com, the average household income is $27,000 (increased from approximately $20,000 in 2010). The reservation continues to have ongoing difficulties with jobs, and the unemployment rate is staggering at 56% (increased from 49% in 2000).[1]

Statistics from the Navajo Epidemiology Study finds that unintentional injury is the primary cause of death on the Navajo Nation (**Table 1**).[2] Alcoholism remains a significant problem on the Navajo Reservation contributing to unintentional injury and death from cirrhosis of the liver, which is the fifth leading cause of death (behind injury, cancer, heart disease, and diabetes). Suicide rates are high and the seventh leading cause of death. Approximately one in four smoke. Substance abuse, obesity, and depression rates are significantly greater than those of the general US population.

VOLUNTEERING IN GALLUP, NEW MEXICO AND CHINLE, ARIZONA

Following my introduction to the Navajo Peoples, I was informed that there was an existing hand surgery clinic run by Ms Andra Battocchio (certified hand therapist) in Chinle, Arizona. The clinic was founded by Dr Charlie Hamlin, from Denver, and

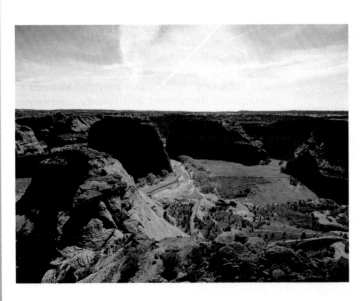

Fig. 1. A view of Canyon De Chelley National Monument from the top of the trail leading to the white house.

Table 1
Causes of death at the Navajo Nation

Rank	Cause of Death	Count	Rate per 100,000	Percent of All Deaths[a]
1	Unintentional injuries	752	107.73	18.9
2	Cancer	506	72.49	12.7
3	Heart disease[b]	485	69.48	12.2
4	Diabetes	228	32.66	5.7
5	Chronic liver disease and cirrhosis	224	32.09	5.6
6	Influenza and pneumonia	181	25.93	4.6
7	Suicide	119	17.05	3.0
8	Stroke	107	15.33	2.7
9	Septicemia	90	12.89	2.3
10	Dementia	84	12.03	2.1
11	Assault	83	11.89	2.1
12	Alcohol dependence syndrome	81	11.60	2.0
13	Renal failure	77	11.03	1.9
14	Hypertensive disease	59	8.45	1.5
15	Chronic obstructive pulmonary disease	49	7.02	1.2

[a] Percent based on known cause (n = 3975).
[b] Heart disease includes: chronic rheumatic heart disease, ischemic heart disease, pulmonary heart disease, and International Classification of Diseases-10 classifications of "other forms of heart disease."
From Foley, D, Kinlacheeny, JB, Yazzie, D. Navajo Nation Mortality Report, 2006-2009: Arizona and New Mexico Data. Navajo Epidemiology Center. 2009. Available at: http://www.nec.navajo-nsn.gov/Portals/0/Reports/Vital%20 Statistics%20Report%202006%20to%202009%20FINAL. pdf.

Andra, back in the mid-1990s at the Chinle Comprehensive Health Care Facility (**Fig. 3**). Charlie described the founding of the clinic after meeting with Navajo leadership, and the rationale for choosing Chinle for a location was because of its central location on the reservation and (in part) its proximity to Canyon De Chelley.[3] The hand clinic began in June 1994 and it continues to this day. Andra creates an annual schedule of clinics at 3- to 4-week intervals and willing volunteer hand surgeons from all over the country select dates that they are able come. She is incredible and maintains a tireless devotion for her patients and for the hand clinic. Without Andra there simply

is no hand clinic. When I began volunteering and up to recently, Charlie was still coming once or twice per year. He has since retired.

Shortly following my initiation into the Chinle, I had another serendipitous event where I was speaking with Dr Samuel Chun, a good friend and former Mayo Hand Fellow. He practices in Santa Fe, New Mexico. Samuel is an extraordinary individual. He is an exceptional surgeon and human being, giving of himself quietly and without notoriety. Meeting and getting to know him and his wife, Sarah, over the years has been one of the highlights of my career. Samuel coined the phrase: "You don't have to travel far to find people in need." He mentioned that he happened to work a hand surgery clinic in Gallup, New Mexico at their Indian health service (IHS) hospital and that he could use a partner to help run a hand clinic in perpetuity, in a similar fashion as the Chinle Clinic. We established monthly clinics where we would come on alternate months. In contrast to Chinle, the Gallup IHS hospital is the largest in the country and has dedicated orthopedists (**Fig. 4**). At the time I was introduced to the Gallup Indian Medical Center, Dr Randolph Copeland was head of orthopedic surgery. Like Samuel, Randy is an extraordinary individual and has also deeply inspired and influenced me. In a government-run system where resources are limited, it is difficult to recruit and maintain dedicated orthopedic surgeons and maintain the highest level of care available for patients. No one could do it better than Randy. His quiet dedication and perseverance in overcoming hurdle after hurdle on a daily basis was inspirational. The staff and patients understandably loved him. Reflective of his understated accomplishments, I really did not appreciate how impressive Randy was as a leader until he stepped down as chief. Samuel has since also retired from coming to Gallup and I sorely miss our routine correspondence.

THE LOGISTICS OF VOLUNTEERING AT THE RESERVATION

Anyone who has worked in a government-run hospital can appreciate the challenges associated with credentialing and caring for patients in the system. For a typical surgeon with a type A personality, it requires tempered expectations. When I was on staff at Duke, I worked intimately with the Durham Veterans Administration Medical Center, so my expectations were (I thought) appropriately tempered. However, the IHS aspires to function at the level of a Veterans Administration. Volunteers are scrutinized by the system to the same level of employees. There is a lot of

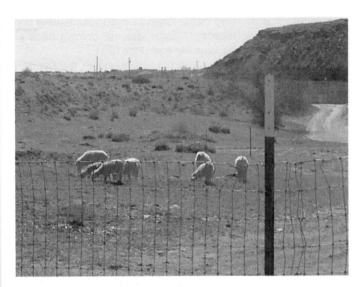

Fig. 2. A flock of sheep along the roadside.

paperwork that is necessary to be credentialed. And like credentialing at any health care facility that one works for, it requires updating every 2 years. In addition, the government requires recurring fingerprinting and background checks for individuals. Things often move slowly and often only to then require immediate attention.

One of the major recent issues associated with outreach for the IHS has been malpractice coverage. When I first began volunteering at the reservation, the understanding was that volunteers were covered, like Veterans Administration Medical Centers, by tort reform. However, although this applies to employees of the IHS, volunteers and contractors have ironically recently been separated out. Some of us are fortunate enough to have coverage from our home institutions. However, as

one may imagine, this is a sticking point for individuals who do not have that coverage. This problem has forced a 4-month pause in the Chinle hand clinic, which has now just recently restarted with individuals who have their own coverage for now until, it is hoped, a final solution is accomplished.

One of the nice features of volunteering at the IHS is that the government reimburses your travel expenses (or at least most of them). But it also is nuanced. Although years ago they were similar, Chinle and Gallup facilities have different systems of reimbursement for flights, hotels, and car rentals. Chinle currently requires surgeons to go through a process of becoming a contractor with the federal government, called the system for awards management (SAM). Individuals go to a Web site and create a DUNS number, which is linked to an

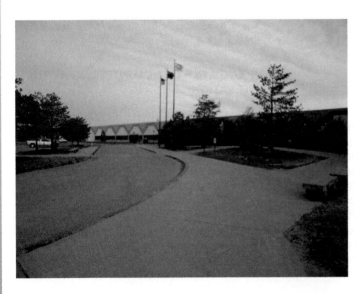

Fig. 3. Chinle Comprehensive Health Care Facility. It has approximately 60 beds and the medical staff includes: family physicians, internists, pediatricians, general surgeons, obstetricians/gynecologists, anesthesiologists, and a psychiatrist.

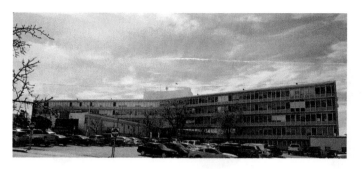

Fig. 4. Gallup Indian Medical Center. It is one of the busiest Indian health service hospitals in the United States with 99 beds and four operating rooms. There is a full-time orthopedic staff with three to six orthopedic surgeons on staff at a given time.

account that they deposit reimbursement for travel. Gallup continues to simply write a check for reimbursement directly to you after you submit receipts. They each have advantages and disadvantages. The SAM system gives the provider flexibility to arrange your own flights and typically reimburses fully. The more traditional system used in Gallup arranges the flights for you (based on the airline they have a relationship with) and reimburses hotel (up to a certain amount) and car rentals. You can use the government rate for hotels and this can help with the costs for some chains. The SAM system requires a significant amount of time to navigate the approval process and needs to be renewed annually. Thankfully the Chinle hand clinic staff is helpful in guiding us through the process.

The Chinle hand clinic typically runs from Wednesday through Friday. Wednesday consists of a full-day clinic. On Thursdays, there are surgeries in the morning, followed by a clinic in the afternoon. All of Friday is a surgical day. In Gallup, I typically go over a period of 2 days: Thursday clinic and Friday surgery. Although stressful at first, the inability to personally follow patients postoperatively, took some getting used to. However, follow-up care is reliably performed by the therapists in Chinle, and an orthopedist or the physician's assistant in Gallup. It is easy for them to call if there are questions or concerns following surgery. And they welcome us checking in on how patients are recovering. In addition, if a patient needs to see a hand surgeon following surgery, a subsequent hand clinic is forthcoming in 3 to 4 weeks.

One of the keys to the success and longevity of the clinics is that there is the continuity of care. Having a regular reliable clinic in the near future helps provide consistent and optimal care for the patients. It helps earn the respect of the medical system and loyalty of our patients. In addition, the presence of a consistent advocate for the clinic with "boots on the ground" is essential. Andra has been that person for many years in Chinle. Her consistent energy and presence drives the clinic. In Gallup, Gerilene is the nurse in the orthopedic clinic who coordinates the hand surgery clinic

and visits. Without her help, we would be lost. I have learned to appreciate all of the things that go on behind the scenes to make these clinics run, which we volunteers often take for granted.

Although I think the current structure for volunteerism is good, there remain some challenges with the current system. Having a clinic on one day with surgery the following day can burden patients to come twice in 2 days. We had discussed the possibility of clinic in the morning and surgery that same afternoon. But depending on the operating room availability and staffing, the amount of surgical time can be compromised to the point where it is less efficient than an all-day clinic followed by a full surgical day. In addition, many patients have diabetes and having them fast until the afternoon is problematic.

THE PRACTICE

Although both facilities have the usual bread and butter hand surgery cases and patients, there are some differences. Because the hospital has a dedicated orthopedic staff, Gallup tends to be a general orthopedic and trauma referral center. This attracts more complex trauma, pediatric patients, and larger overall volume of patients. Neglected trauma, such as malunion/nonunion of fractures and their sequelae, are common. Hand burns are also commonly seen because many on the reservation depend on burning wood for heat. Also, because many conditions and injuries are neglected, there is a high incidence of infection and complications related to prior infection. Congenital anomalies of the hand are also not uncommon and include supernumery digits, congenital absence of the thumb (**Fig. 5**), and congenital trigger thumbs. Associated with the high rate of diabetes, there is a significant number of patients with compressive/peripheral neuropathy and trigger fingers. Interestingly, I have seen a substantial amount of rheumatoid arthritis over the years. Because access to rheumatology and antirheumatoid medication is difficult, these conditions are often poorly controlled (**Fig. 6**).

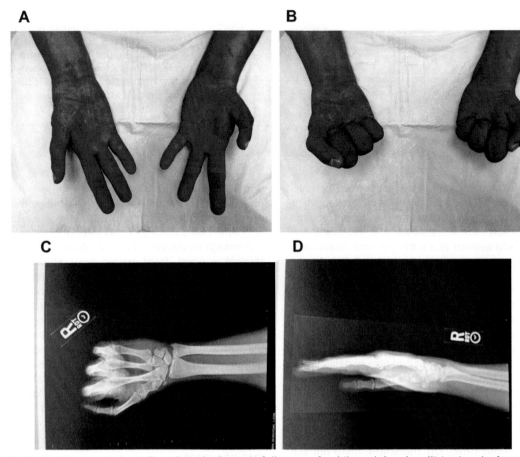

Fig. 5. (*A*, *B*) A man in the Gallup Clinic I had seen in follow-up after bilateral thumb pollicizations in the remote past. (*C*) Anteroposterior and (*D*) lateral radiographs of the right side.

Chinle has a more predictable and consistent presence of hand therapy and access to special studies, such as electromyography. Gallup has to send patients to a private hospital in Gallup, Rehoboth Medical Center, for special studies and procedures, which requires special approval from leadership and is considered on a case-by-case basis. Fortunately, both facilities have access to ultrasonography, although not readily available for us to use in the clinics. Patients must be sent to radiology for these studies. Gallup has a dedicated pathologist, whereas all pathology specimens must be sent out from Chinle.

The clinics help set up the operating room cases for the week. Patients considered to be surgical candidates are seen in the morning clinic. If the surgeon and patient decide surgery is appropriate, they are scheduled. Many patients in clinic are there for injections and clinical decision-making. Unfortunately, because transportation and communication are difficult for many Navajo, the rate of clinic no-shows has traditionally been high. Once surgery has been decided on, medical clearance is to be performed by the volunteer or the patient's primary care provider.

Gallup has four operating rooms and Chinle has two. The anesthesiologists are generally very good. The staff is often willing to stay late when we have a large number of cases. When indicated, admitting patients for overnight stay following surgery requires coordination in Gallup with one of the orthopedic surgeons and, in Chinle, with one of the general surgeons.

LESSONS LEARNED

There were also cultural nuances that I had to get used to. I learned, over time, to talk less and listen more when interviewing patients. At first, I was not sure if patients understood, so I tended to try and say the same thing several different ways. In retrospect, most fully understood what I was saying and explaining/proposing to them. Silence during conversation seems acceptable with most Navajo people. I find that I am learning to accept silence between statements in my

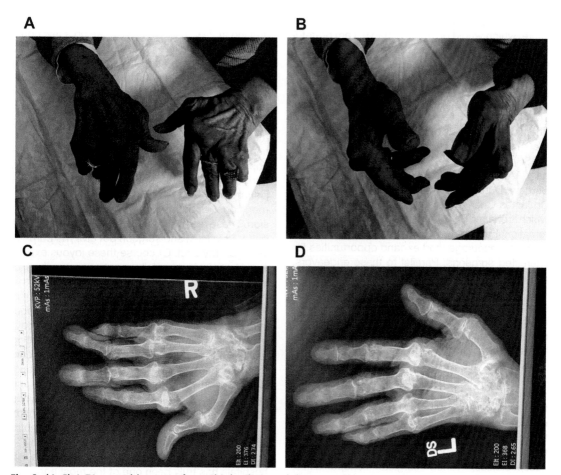

Fig. 6. (*A, B*) A 71-year-old woman from Chinle Clinic with long-standing rheumatoid arthritis. (*C*) Right and (*D*) left anteroposterior radiographs demonstrate the severe arthritic changes and deformity.

personal practice as well. Like many things, it takes time to earn people's trust, but I found that there is a general willingness, if not eagerness, to want to trust us as caregivers. In addition, these patients have been some of the most appreciative patients who I have been fortunate enough to help care for.

Being flexible is an important part of the experience of volunteering at the reservation. Equipment for cases is hit or miss and one must learn to improvise and be flexible with respect to methods and surgical techniques. These experiences have helped me evolve into a better surgeon and expand ideas of how to get things accomplished. When in doubt, I have erred on immobilizing longer, and being generally more conservative postoperatively, especially in Gallup where therapy access is less predictable. I have learned to solicit equipment from companies that I can bring when I travel to the reservation and use for surgery. I was impressed at how willing folks, such as the Synthes

representative, were in providing whatever they can to help. However, this practice has become more difficult over the years because of regulations.

Being willing to help in any capacity possible has helped me as a surgeon and to gain the respect of the staff and patients. I have helped surgeons with nonhand cases, such as tibial plateau and ankle fractures, on numerous occasions in Gallup. I have helped the Chinle obstetrics/gynecology doctors with removal of implanted birth control devices. I have learned to resist the temptation to say "that is not my job" or "that is not my problem." Beyond the joy of helping for its own sake, this spirit of "what can I do to help" gives the volunteer street credibility.

The experience of volunteering has also been humbling to me, in a beautiful way. Many of the (especially neglected) conditions are not typically seen in most medical centers where resources and access are so readily available. Often times I was unsure of the best approach for these neglected maladies/conditions. The providers in the trenches would often have experience to share, which would be most valuable. I am grateful to have had these experiences, which have helped (and continue to help) make me a better surgeon.

MOVING FORWARD

Over the last 2 to 3 years, there has been increased attention to domestic and international outreach by the American Society for Surgery of the Hand (ASSH), The American Academy of Orthopedic Surgery (AAOS), and the American Association of Hand Surgery. During his presidential year of the ASSH, Dr James Chang formed an outreach committee, which is chaired by Dr Don Lalonde and includes international and domestic divisions. The aim is to support, encourage, and expand opportunities for interested surgeons. Parallel to these endeavors, president of the AAOS Board of Specialties, Dr Amy Ladd, a regular volunteer at the Chinle hand clinic, highlighted outreach at the IHS and created a taskforce with similar aims of increasing awareness and facilitating participation of interested orthopedic surgeons in varied subspecialties.

It has been incredible to learn how many physicians and surgeons, in their own quiet way, are performing outreach of some kind in all areas of the country. Many are linked to groups that have considerable memberships and diversity of expertise. The promise of expanding access beyond orthopedic surgery into internal medicine and subspecialties, varied surgical subspecialties, and just about any areas of medicine it is hoped can someday be realized.

There are many reservations and other groups of individuals for whom the needs are as great as those of the Navajo. There are numerous reservations with woefully inadequate and understaffed facilities or no facilities at all. Depending on the infrastructure and surgeon interest, the possibility of a system that has varied location options and more date options may allow interested individuals to experience the joy of volunteering in more convenient locations to their home. A dedicated system with a large enough group could expand to outreach beyond the Native American population and to other groups in need in the United States.

SUMMARY

Oftentimes as I approach the scheduled trips to the reservation, things are crazy busy at my practice and I feel like I am pulled 50 different ways. The week before the trip I am sheepishly apologizing to my wife and daughter that I will be going away (again). I catch myself looking on it as a distraction and added stressor, regularly traveling the night following a busy clinic/operating room day and arriving at 2 AM to the hotel to wake up a few hours later and start clinic and go through the hectic week. All too often I have muttered to myself that this is too much and not sustainable.

The voice in my head then asks: "Marco, where do you find your joy?" I realize then that not going was never an option and it is always about how to make it work. The joy comes of learning from patients, examining them, understanding their condition, and offering treatment options and partnering with them on their journey. Giving not just my knowledge and technical skill, but also humor, hope, empathy, care, sympathy, and compassion. These repeated exercises not only make me a better physician and surgeon but give me purpose and feed my soul. Of course these joyous experiences occur in our daily practice, regardless of where we work. However, I would argue that this ritual is done in its most special and purest form in the setting of volunteerism. No distractions about insurance coverage, no conflict related to payments, no motivations beyond the joy of wanting to help. Dr Paul Brand stated these sentiments most eloquently in the 1991 ASSH Annual Meeting: "When we have shared not only our knowledge and skill but part of ourselves with our patients, when something of our hope and faith awaken in them, then something comes back to us. It is in the mutuality of medical care that we experience real joy."[4]

My experience with domestic outreach at the IHS hospitals has truly been one of the most enriching experiences of my career and life. I have received much more than I could give. I feel blessed to have had the opportunity to visit with, share, and help, in whatever way I can, the patients of Gallup and Chinle. I sincerely thank the many people, such as Andra, Charlie, Gerilene, Samuel, and Randy, who helped facilitate this wonderful experience for me. I encourage anyone reading this to consider domestic outreach and remember Dr Samuel Chun: "You don't have to travel far to find people in need."

REFERENCES

1. Discover Navajo fact sheet. 2010 US Census Data. Available at: https://www.discovernavajo.com/factsheet.aspx.
2. Foley D, Kinlacheeny JB, Yazzie D. Navajo Nation mortality report, 2006-2009. Window Rock (AZ): Navajo Epidemiology Center; 2009.
3. Hamlin C. Volunteerism on the Navajo reservation: the Chinle hand service. Clin Orthop Relat Res 2002;(396):36–42.
4. Brand PW. The pursuit of happiness. J Hand Surg Am 1992;17(4):593–7.

Guidelines for Short-Term Hand Surgery Outreach Trips
Building Trust and Establishing Continuity

Fraser J. Leversedge, MD[a,b,c,d],*

KEYWORDS

- Hand surgery • Outreach • Mission • Global health • Medical volunteer • Touching hands project
- Honduras

KEY POINTS

- The goals and scope of a medical brigade should be established through healthy communication with the host institution. Careful understanding as to local needs and available resources facilitate reasonable expectations for the medical team, patients, and local community.
- Flexibility is the key to any mission. Meticulous planning, particularly in conjunction with local contacts, reduces inherent risks of travel, transportation of supplies, and personal safety. Potential fluctuations in local circumstances (politics, economy, social order, and so forth) or a lack of expected resources should be considered.
- Although short-term goals associated with direct patient care are a focus, investing in the education of the local medical team is vital for the development of competencies that may permit the gradual transition of patient care to local surgeons and other medical providers, such as hand therapists. This supports the concept that "teaching a person to fish will feed them for a lifetime."
- Developing strategies for the continuity of patient care improves overall satisfaction and patient outcomes, in particular, reducing risk of unforeseen complications or noncompliance with treatment.
- Creating time and space for reflection is invaluable for all team members. Personal growth is inevitable, but its impact should be processed and shared with others to be of greatest benefit.

INTRODUCTION

Prior to this, our journey, I felt like I was stuck in an eddy like a leaf going round and round and round while this enormous river of life flowed past. But your cumulative life's energy, laughter and camaraderie released me back into that powerful river of life and once again you guys made me feel alive and productive to our strange world. We created, for a week, our own little Woodstock. A happening. Thanks. You guys are swell. See ya (Participant, Touching Hands Project–Honduras).

Providing high-quality care for conditions affecting the hand and upper limb in low-income and middle-income countries has been a goal of numerous outreach organizations, emphasized in

Disclosure Statement: The author has nothing to disclose pertinent to the subject matter of the article.
[a] Plastic Surgery, Duke University, Durham, NC, USA; [b] Touching Hands Project, San Pedro Sula, Honduras; [c] American Foundation for Surgery of the Hand, Chicago, IL, USA; [d] Department of Orthopaedic Surgery, Duke University, DUMC Box 2836, Durham, NC 27710, USA
* Department of Orthopaedic Surgery, Duke University, DUMC Box 2836, Durham, NC 27710.
E-mail address: fraser.leversedge@duke.edu

Hand Clin 35 (2019) 449–455
https://doi.org/10.1016/j.hcl.2019.07.008
0749-0712/19/© 2019 Elsevier Inc. All rights reserved.

the United States in 2014 by the creation of the Touching Hands Project under the direction of the American Society for Surgery of the Hand.[1,2] International and domestic outreach efforts in hand surgery have integrated models of other specialties to deliver care, with short-term trips a common form of support.

Recognizing the variations in scope of individual mission trips, it is important to develop both organizational and site-specific short-term and long-term strategies. Four models describing outreach strategies have shaped the purpose and outcomes of mission trips[1]: (1) a direct supply or vertical approach that may be best suited to humanitarian disaster responses; (2) a reverse fellowship model that supports the training of local specialists in a higher-income country; (3) a horizontal approach that primarily provides development support for infrastructure and health care systems; and (4) a diagonal development model that integrates the immediate benefits of the vertical approach with the longer-term strategies of the horizontal approach, encouraging needs-driven patient selection, multispecialty care, bilateral approach to education, and development of infrastructure that encourages a sustainable system for growth of the field in the host country.[3,4] It has been suggested that this diagonal model may be considered ideal; the guidelines for short-term hand surgery trips highlight this vision for high-quality multidisciplinary care, bilateral engagement, and sustainable development.[3]

Effective communication facilitates the success of an independent mission and the growth of a long-term vision. Guidelines are developed through collaboration between organizational and site-specific leadership as well as local hospital and physician leaders and may be considered as (1) planning: premission; (2) on-site: active mission; and (3) postmission. Many of these guidelines overlap in regard to their implementation; however, this general structure should assist in improving outcomes and minimizing risks of the outreach experience.

PLANNING: PREMISSION
Site Selection

The site selection process for an outreach organization is instrumental in promoting a greater vision but is critical for optimizing opportunities for success and for minimizing risk. Often, potential sites present through known connections, such as personal relationships, business contacts, religious organizations, and previous experiences; however, a thorough review of the host institution, the location, and the potential alignment with an outreach organization's mission and vision statements is imperative. Considerations for site selection should include the following.

Needs assessment

A needs assessment of a potential mission site is essential at many levels and is facilitated by communications between the outreach group and the host institution. Understanding the local patient population, the availability and experience of the local medical community, and the medical conditions with which they need the greatest assistance help to shape the effort.[5] It is critical to assess barriers to successful outcomes, such as language or cultural issues, cost, medical care access, and opportunities for continuity of care—both locally and with subsequent mission trips. Discussions with local surgeons who would provide premission patient screening and referrals as well as postoperative care provide important perspective as to a needs-assessment and to perioperative resources; developing a strong relationship with local surgeons based on mutual trust and respect greatly influences the success of an outreach program.

Determining resources

Resources should be considered both for nonclinical and clinical purposes. Nonclinical resources are supportive of the overall mission and include team safety and security, team health and well-being, ground transportation, lodging, and meals. Establishing an experienced local point of contact is essential for coordinating these resources. Clinical resources have a direct and indirect impact on patient care and include previsit patient screening, clinic staffing, interpreters (if applicable), medical record keeping, radiology equipment, surgical resources, and postsurgical care. Other factors, such as a reliable electrical and oxygen supply, modern anesthesia equipment, and laboratory services (including availability of blood or blood products), should be evaluated.

Setting expectations

Setting reasonable expectations assists in determining the suitability of a potential site, particularly if patient needs can be met not only by the visiting surgeon but by the resources available for appropriate perioperative care. Each brigade may have a unique collective skill set and accompanying resources and, therefore, team and local expectations should be adjusted for each trip. Complex procedures (microvascular surgery, free tissue transfer, limb-lengthening procedures, and so forth) may be challenging without patient and local staff/physician education; preparation dictates the timing and introduction of these types of procedures and, therefore, a delay in performing the procedure to a subsequent brigade may be advised in the absence of adequate resources. Strategies for addressing adverse outcomes (infection, failure of procedure, and limb-threatening or life-threatening conditions) should be considered also, based on perceived challenges with language and cultural barriers, the relative risk of surgical interventions, and the potential for noncompliance.

Establishing effective communications

The successful development of an outreach site depends on effective communications. An organizational leader or administrator and a site leader designated by the organization should be accessible for the local institution and local surgeons. Determining optimal methods for communicating information surrounding patient care facilitates effective decision making about new or established patients and for determining resource allocation, such as implant or instrument needs for future cases. As an outreach clinic matures, opportunities for shared and accessible (patient privacy compliant) medical records may improve patient care.

Team Preparation

Team composition and selection

Bringing together a diverse group of individuals, from different specialties and from different places, and creating a high-functioning team in a short period of time are potentiated by the energy and enthusiasm for the mission and the inspiration of helping others in need. The composition of a team and its selection process, however, need to be considered carefully by a team leader and the organization. A mission trip serves a community and its patients and the multispecialty team should be composed of individuals who, collectively, are able to provide the highest level of care for the conditions that are being treated and to serve as ambassadors for the organization. The trip may serve, also, to educate younger surgeons or trainees; however, no individual should practice outside of the scope of experience or level of training because this may endanger patients and the reputation of the mission. A needs assessment should help identify the optimal scope of practice and the skills required to accomplish the expectations of the trip. Also, decisions may be guided by budgetary or financial considerations. The team leader should seek to staff a trip that not only provides a balanced clinical, educational, and cultural experience for each team member but also satisfies the required elements for patient safety and quality care.

Each organization should provide eligibility criteria and guidance for the team leader involved in the selection of team members, including information from previous volunteer evaluations, where applicable. Often, a team that includes both members with previous outreach experience (particularly at the same site) and members embarking on their first mission provides a balance and encourages growth in outreach participation.

Mission and vision statements

The mission and vision statements of the organization should be reviewed by all team members. Individuals may have personal reasons for participating on a mission trip; however, all participants should honor the notion that they are serving something bigger than the individual and be reminded of the collective purpose of the mission trip.

Team introductions

Prior to departure, team introductions may be achieved through 1 or more conference calls and shared e-mails. These communications improve general awareness of the personalities and experiences of those participating on the trip and may lead to the coordination of travel, equipment and supply management/transportation, and lodging plans.

Review of team and individual goals

As part of initial communications, the team leader may provide an overview of the team composition and encourage discussion as to individual members' goals for the trip. This baseline assessment of individual goals is purposeful because it permits team members to reflect on their experiences during daily debriefings during the week and at the end of the trip.

Site and schedule overview

A review of the local hospital/clinic and the pertinent aspects of the trip improves preparedness of the team and provides team members with awareness of expectations for the brigade. Providing suggestions for packing (clothing, personal items, personal health, and so forth), dietary considerations, and local electronic and telephone use can be helpful, particularly because the availability of replacement items may be limited.

Safety

Safety is critical to the success, and sustainability, of an outreach program. All outreach programs should review and communicate safety-related concerns and strategies for mitigating risk for individuals and for the team.

Several aspects of safety include the following:

- International travel—the US Department of State advisory Web site provides information about international destinations: https://travel.state.gov/content/travel/en/traveladvisories/traveladvisories.html.
- Local travel—local travel is best organized through the officially recognized local group contact.
- Health—international outreach often occurs in regions that have endemic health risks. The Centers for Disease Control and Prevention Web site provides health information for international destinations: https://wwwnc.cdc.gov/travel/destinations/list.
- Safety in numbers—many safety risks are minimized by using common sense and careful communication strategies. Travel in groups and with local guides or security reduces exposure to risk and individual travel.

Travel guidelines

Travel policies, such as flight and lodging instructions, baggage allowance, shipping of supplies, and visas, should be reviewed and reinforced in the months leading up to the trip. Passport expiration dates relative to the travel return date should be checked by all team members well in advance of the trip to avoid restrictions on travel and last-minute disappointment.

Setting expectations, reinforcing policies, and seeking input

A majority of organizational policies involve team safety, conduct, and patient care and, therefore, these should be reviewed with all team members such that the policies are supportive of the team goals and not perceived as adversarial or restrictive. In advance of the trip, assigning responsibilities to team members improves expectations and improves engagement in and promotion of leadership activities. It is critical to engage all team members with a spirit of intentional leadership for all aspects of the mission; prompt feedback from all team members, including constructive criticism, promotes a healthy environment for the entire team.[6]

ON-SITE: ACTIVE MISSION
Team Building

The meeting place—team arrivals

Although individual locations vary, establishing a routine for team member arrivals ensures that the team and supplies arrive together and the team can navigate immigrations and customs as a group—sometimes with the assistance of local contacts. It reinforces the collective nature of the

brigade and it provides an opportunity for team members to meet.

Introductions—team-building activities

On arrival, there are often numerous tasks that require attention prior to the start of clinical activities; however, creating time for a group activity enhances awareness as to the local environment and promotes personal interactions. This team-building activity can take the form of a hike, a roundtable interactive discussion, and/or a group dinner.

Assigning roles and responsibilities

Prior to travel, certain responsibilities may be delegated to individual team members in order to permit preparation for the clinical and nonclinical tasks associated with the brigade. Organizational activities, such as blogs or photo documentation, may be overlooked if no one is assigned this responsibility. Delegation of duties for both running the clinic and preparing and coordinating the operating rooms includes patient documentation (charting, photo and/or video documentation, and so forth), scheduling of cases, medical clearance, confirmation of implant availability, and patient education. Unpacking and taking inventory of supplies and instruments are critical to the efficient delivery of care during the mission.

Collective wisdom

Team building is a process that continues over the course of a mission. Team members should be encouraged to actively contribute because the collective wisdom of the group maximizes the experiences and outcomes of the team as a whole.

Organizational Excellence

Integration

It is critical for team members to integrate into the team, sometimes stepping out of a comfort zone or routine. Similarly, the brigade must integrate with the local institution's system and processes. Often, a recognition of differences or variations in these processes may improve care through reconciliation—this might be related to the details of the time-out process, patient consent and education, or clinical documentation.

Resource management

Recognizing resource limitations and the importance of careful surgical planning influences the daily and weekly schedule regarding case indications and selection. Simple processes, such as instrument sterilization and the confirmation of implant availability, may determine case order and resource allocation. Communication with the entire staff (local and outreach teams) minimizes the risks of case cancellations, wasted resources, or inappropriate procedures.

Delegation of responsibilities

Organizational excellence requires the active participation and intentional leadership of the entire team, including local participants. The team leader should seek opportunities to delegate responsibilities based on experience to increase accountability and engagement throughout the team member experience levels.

Patient Care

Primum non nocere (first, do no harm)

It is recognized that interventions, such as surgery, carry inherent risks. It is incumbent on the brigade to maintain the highest standards of care to avoid adverse outcomes and to prevent harm. The mission trip is not a place to experiment, to practice outside of the scope of experience, or to abdicate reasonable responsibilities to the patient and the clinical care team.

Consent process

Consent for treatment is the first step in doing no harm and toward optimal outcomes. A careful consent process, including patient identification and the subsequent time-out, involves the shared decision making of a patient and family and the comprehensive review as to the rationale (indications), inherent risks and benefits of the treatment and its alternatives, potential outcomes, and perioperative expectations for the procedure. An interpreter should be involved when indicated.

Daily board rounds

Daily board rounds (a review of the operative cases for the day) integrate many of the critical elements of patient care while on an international mission. They should bring together all members of the greater team—outreach and local providers, including surgeons, nurses, trainees, therapists, and anesthesia staff, with a complete review of the day's schedule. This process can improve interdisciplinary communication, avoid wrong-site or wrong-type surgery, reduce resource inefficiencies, improve anesthesia care, and coordinate the perioperative care of the patients, such as implant choices and postsurgery rehabilitation plans.

Transfer of care

Patient care involves the transfer of care throughout the mission trip, including transfers of care within the team itself and to local surgeons and therapists once the brigade has departed. Communication is essential. This may take the form of chart documentation in clinic that outlines the surgical and anesthesia plan or an operative note that explains the operative findings, treatment, and postsurgical plans.

Patient education

Outcomes are influenced by a patient's understanding of the condition, the purpose of treatment, and instructions to protect the healing process and to accelerate the recovery process. Education should be confirmed in the patient's native language and resources should be provided to improve the retention of these communications. Preoperative and postoperative rehabilitation instructions are valuable in conjunction with the surgical team, the local surgeon, and therapy.

Continuity of care

Because the brigade may have limited opportunities to educate and to care for patients postoperatively, confirmation as to plans for continuity of treatment with local caregivers is imperative. Restricted transportation options, poor social support, or concerns regarding patient understanding or compliance with treatment may indicate that surgery should be postponed. Outcomes assessments are ensured when patients have follow-up with subsequent brigades.

Documentation

Standards

Maintaining an accessible and legible patient care record is imperative for ensuring patient safety and for documenting and transferring the patient care. Local standards for record archiving supersede forms developed by an outreach organization; however, creating an efficient and reproducible system for use by specialty brigades may be considered and approved by the host institution.

Records: accessible, readable, valuable

Although the electronic medical record represents a standard in the United States, most countries do not have the infrastructure currently to support a secure, accessible electronic medical record. Because the continuity of care for a patient may be delivered by different clinicians—from the same or subsequent brigades, or by local providers—legible and comprehensive documentation of the pertinent clinical assessment, treatment plan, and surgical findings is critical. Integration of clinical photos and videos is advantageous and may be hosted in a digital record, potentially accessible via the Internet, which make the chart portable and accessible, both before and after the outreach trip.

Cultural Sensitivity

Many sources of patient dissatisfaction and misunderstanding are related to cultural insensitivity. A shared decision-making process with patients must consider cultural bias; a lack of recognition or insensitivity to local customs may reduce opportunities to have an impact on care. The global outreach experience provides opportunities for cultural competency training with mentorship.[7]

Education

Education should be emphasized on all mission trips and includes opportunities for the outreach team, for the local clinical providers, and for patients. The outreach team benefits from the cultural exchange and from the bilateral exchange of ideas with local providers. The team should be responsible for educating local surgeons and therapists as to the nature of procedures performed and the postoperative protocols. Reference materials (online or printed references) are always advantageous, and post-trip communications permit ongoing reinforcement of treatment concepts. Internally, the team members have various levels of experience and are able to take advantage of the various backgrounds for meaningful learning opportunities. There are increasing opportunities for integrating international outreach experiences within the framework of formal training program curricula.[8,9]

Patient education is critical for optimizing outcomes and may take the form of improving awareness as to the condition, potential treatment options, and recommendations. Perioperative treatments, including medical management, therapy, and surgical care should be reviewed using appropriate interpretation, learning resources, and follow-up. Education that focuses on injury prevention[10] and occupational safety can be invaluable and can be extended to collaborative efforts with local industry partners.

POSTMISSION
Debriefing

At the completion of each trip, reflections about the experience from all team members should be documented by the team leader and/or organization, along with key points from daily debriefings. These comments influence planning for the next brigade but also the growth of the organization, particularly when feedback is considered in a comprehensive manner. Constructive criticism should be welcomed and feedback from the host site should be encouraged. A critical evaluation of overall patient care, resource utilization, and barriers to success provides enhanced opportunities for future trips.

Quality Improvement

As an extension of the team debriefing, a quality improvement assessment should be completed that considers the complications or adverse outcomes of treatment.[11] These cases, as well as potential near-miss cases where a flaw in a system of care almost leads to an adverse outcome, should be analyzed critically to implement safeguards for future care.

Continuity of Care
Postsurgical care

Effective and timely communication with the local team managing the postoperative care of a patient is essential for continuity of care and, ultimately, for patient outcomes. These principles apply to patients not undergoing surgery but for whom additional assessment or testing is required and for those patients for whom a staged procedure might be warranted. Arrangements for the transition of care from the outreach team to local physicians, surgeons, and therapists should be established prior to the start of the mission trip, and engagement with this local team should be ongoing throughout the trip. Many local surgeons and/or their trainees may participate in patient care throughout the week, which improves awareness as to treatment strategies; however, careful documentation as to the condition, treatment, and postoperative plan should be clear.

Communication strategies

Although direct communication is preferred, postmission communication is expected when there are questions or concerns regarding ongoing patient care. Accessibility, or lack thereof, may be a limiting factor for effective premission and postmission communications and, therefore, establishing a reliable method of communication is imperative. Direct phone communication, e-mail, video links, and Web-based video platforms may serve individual needs. As encrypted and deidentified digital photographs and video become more easily communicated, these resources have improved clinical decision making in conjunction with the local provider.

Management of complications

Strategies for postoperative care and communication, discussed previously, improve timeliness of treatment of postsurgical complications and reduce the impact of noncompliance and/or incomplete recognition of adverse outcomes through the engagement of patient and local provider. Patient and local provider education, greater familiarity with postoperative protocols, and accessibility for perioperative concerns may all have a positive impact on minimizing undesired complications of treatment.

Outreach collaboration efforts

Although there are numerous organizations participating in global health outreach, the coordination of patient care and resources between groups is rare.[12] There is great potential for improving the sharing of information about the timing of upcoming trips, site logistics, local resources, and patient care.

Resource Reassessment and Preparation for Next Visit

Preparation for the next visit and for the longer-term strategy for providing care includes a reassessment of resources, opportunities for greater integration and collaboration with local providers, needs assessment for patient continuity of care and for initiation of new treatment, and cost analysis to determine the relative value of the program and to improve the efficacy and optimal use of appropriate resources during the mission trip.[13,14]

Communication and Goal Setting

Ongoing efforts to improve outreach experiences require individual and organizational commitments to excellence through an active review and reassessment process. Reviews should include communication with and feedback from local hosts, team members, and team leaders. A careful analysis of financial strategies and volunteer engagement permits continued advancement of opportunities for outcomes research, resource development, education, and patient care.

REFERENCES

1. Chung KY. The role for international outreach in hand surgery. J Hand Surg Am 2017;42(8):652–5.
2. The Commission Process. The lancet commission on global surgery. Available at: http://www.lancetglobal surgery.org/#!background/z4c08. 2016. Accessed April 11, 2019.
3. Corlew S, Fan VY. A model for building capacity in international plastic surgery. ReSurge International. Ann Plast Surg 2011;67(6):568–70.
4. Patel PB, Hoyler M, Maine R, et al. An opportunity for diagonal development in global surgery: cleft lip and palate care in resource-limited settings. Plast Surg Int 2012;2012:892437.
5. Nugent AG, Panthaki Z, Thaller S. The planning and execution of surgical hand mission trips in developing countries. J Craniofac Surg 2015;26(4):1055–7.
6. Hargett CW, Doty JP, Hauck JN, et al. Developing a model for effective leadership in healthcare: a concept mapping approach. J Healthc Leadersh 2017;28(9):69–78.
7. Yao CA, Swanson J, McCullough M, et al. The medical mission and modern core competency training: a 10-year follow-up of resident experiences in global plastic surgery. Plast Reconstr Surg 2016;138(3):531e–8e.
8. Knudson MM, Tarpley MJ, Numann PJ. Global surgery opportunities for US surgical residents: an interim report. J Surg Educ 2015;72(4):e60–5.
9. Mackay DR. Obtaining Accreditation Council for Graduate Medical Education approval for international rotations during plastic surgery residency training. J Craniofac Surg 2015;26(4):1086–7.
10. Chung KY, Hanemaayer A, Poenaru D. Pediatric hand surgery in global health: the role for international outreach. Ann Plast Surg 2017;78(2):162–70.
11. Schneider WJ, Politis GD, Gosain AK, et al. Volunteers in plastic surgery guidelines for providing surgical care for children in the less developed world. Plast Reconstr Surg 2011;127:2477–86.
12. Medoff S, Freed J. The ned for formal surgical global health programs and improved mission trip coordination. Ann Glob Health 2016;82(4):634–8.
13. Nolte MT, Maroukis BL, Chung KC, et al. A systemic review of economic analysis of surgical mission trips using the World Health Organization criteria. World J Surg 2016;40(8):1874–84.
14. Qiu X, Nasser JS, Sue GR, et al. Cost-effectiveness analysis of humanitarian hand surgery trips according to WHO-CHOICE thresholds. J Hand Surg Am 2019;44(2):93–103.

Upper Extremity Burns in the Developing World
A Neglected Epidemic

Sarah E. Sasor, MD[a],*, Kevin C. Chung, MD, MS[b]

KEYWORDS

- Hand burns • Burn care in low income countries • Global burn care • Burn epidemiology
- Hand burn rehabilitation • Scar contracture • Burn reconstruction • Hand reconstruction

KEY POINTS

- The majority of burns occur in low- and middle-income countries, where access to basic health care is limited.
- The upper extremity is involved in more than 80% of burns. Delayed, inappropriate, or inadequate treatment of upper extremity burns causes severe disability.
- Many burn survivors face extreme poverty as the result of functional impairment, loss of employment, and poor public support.
- Much of burn-related suffering can be prevented through education, simple interventions, and basic care.

INTRODUCTION

Burns are devastating injuries that cause significant morbidity, emotional distress, and decreased quality of life. Advances in care have improved survival and functional outcomes over the last several decades; however, burns remain a major public health problem in developing countries. Globally, more than 11 million people seek medical attention for burns each year.[1] Burns are among the leading causes of death and disability worldwide.[2,3]

The burden of burn injury falls predominantly on the poor. More than 95% of burns occur in low- and middle-income countries (LMIC), where education, safety regulations, prevention programs, and access to basic health care are lacking.[4] Treatment is often delayed, inappropriate, or inadequate. Follow-up is problematic and rehabilitation services are nonexistent. The sequelae of untreated and undertreated burns are often severe enough to cause permanent disability. In developing countries, this can mean unemployment, family abandonment, social segregation, and extreme poverty.

Although each hand accounts for only 3% of total body surface area, they are involved in more than 80% of severe burns.[5] Appropriate treatment of upper extremity burns is a priority; even small burns to the hand can result in severe functional disability. Scarring, joint contractures, stiffness, and chronic pain are devastating in the upper extremity owing to the dependence on hand function for productivity and financial independence.

The purpose of this article is to review upper extremity burn epidemiology, risk factors, prevention strategies, and treatment options in resource-limited settings.

Disclosure Statement: This work was supported by a Midcareer Investigator Award in Patient-Oriented Research (2 K24-AR053120–06) to K.C. Chung. The content is solely the responsibility of the authors and does not necessarily represent the official views of the National Institutes of Health.

[a] Department of Plastic Surgery, Medical College of Wisconsin, Milwaukee, WI, USA; [b] Department of Surgery, Section of Plastic Surgery, University of Michigan, 1500 East Medical Center Drive, 2130 Taubman Center, SPC 5340, Ann Arbor, MI 48109, USA
* Corresponding author.
E-mail address: ssasor@gmail.com

Hand Clin 35 (2019) 457–466
https://doi.org/10.1016/j.hcl.2019.07.010

EPIDEMIOLOGY

National and public health registries, hospital data, community surveys, and a variety of additional sources are used to gather information on burn epidemiology. The accuracy and availability of these data varies considerably. Most published literature characterizing the etiology, severity, risk factors, and outcomes of burns is based on populations of patients treated at burn centers. Patients treated in primary care facilities, rural settings, or at home represent a large portion of injuries and often go unaccounted for. This section presents available information on burn epidemiology.

Incidence

Burns are the fourth most common cause of injury worldwide, after traffic accidents, falls, and interpersonal violence.[1] More than 30 million people are affected each year. Although 300,000 deaths are caused by burns and fires annually, the vast majority of burn injuries are not fatal.[4]

The overall incidence of acute burns and prevalence of chronic sequelae have both decreased since 1990.[6] This is attributed to legislative changes, widespread prevention strategies, increased workplace safety, and improved guidelines for referral to burn centers in the developed world.[7] Demographic changes since 1990, including longer life expectancy and a shift in the age distribution toward an older populace, accentuate this decline. The incidence of burns in the developing world remains alarmingly high.[8] Regional variations in social, political, and environmental factors, discussed elsewhere in this article, result in an unequal worldwide distribution.

Morbidity and Sequelae

Nonfatal burns are a leading cause of prolonged hospitalization, chronic pain, disfigurement, and disability. Patients with burns typically benefit from long-term therapy and may require multiple reconstructive procedures to facilitate recovery. In the developing world, resources and access to care are limited. Patients travel long distances for treatment, making follow-up care impractical or impossible. Many survivors receive no further medical services after discharge. Undertreated extremity burns result in severe contractures.

It is estimated that more than 18 million people currently live with the sequelae of hand burns.[9] Many face lifelong disability and extreme poverty as the result of functional impairment and loss of vocational capacity. Social and financial support services are rare in developing countries.

Burden of Disease

The direct cost of medical care varies widely throughout the world. Burn care is generally expensive owing to long hospital stays, specialized dressings, multiple surgeries, and the need for intensive care in severe injuries. In the United States, inpatient care costs $3000 to $5000 per day.[4] Mean total cost of care over a patient's lifetime is $88,218 in high-income countries.[10] Indirect costs, such as lost wages, travel, and costs related to emotional and physical rehabilitation, contribute significantly to the overall economic impact of disease.

The disability-adjusted life-year (DALY) is a metric commonly used to quantify the harmful effect of an injury or disease. Introduced in the World Development Report in 1993, DALY is the sum of the years of life lost (YLL) and years of life lived with disability.[11,12] Burns are among the leading causes of DALYs lost in LMIC.[4] Although burns decrease an individual's overall life expectancy, years of life lived with disability contributes more to DALY calculations for upper extremity burns.

RISK FACTORS

More than 80% of severe burns involve the upper extremity. Hands are generally exposed, used in protective reflexes, and most likely to come into contact with hot substances, chemicals, electrical current, and moving parts (friction). This section reviews risk factors for burn injury.

Socioeconomic

Burns disproportionately affect the poor. More than 95% of burn injuries occur in low- and middle-income regions.[4] Southeast Asia, the Eastern Mediterranean, and Africa have the highest rates of burn mortality worldwide. Even in high-income counties, individuals living in areas of deprivation are more likely to suffer severe burns requiring hospitalization.[7,13] Inferior quality of housing; the absence of preventive devices such as smoke detectors, sprinklers, hot water temperature regulators; and increased rates of smoking, drug, and alcohol abuse in low-income areas place these communities at risk.[14,15]

Race and Ethnicity

In the United States, the rate of nonfatal burns is 122 per 100,000 in black Americans versus 91 per 100,000 in white non-Hispanics.[16] The age-adjusted death rate from burns is also highest in blacks (1.6 per 100,000) compared with American Indians (1.4), Caucasians (0.9), and Asians (0.3).[17] Studies show similar trends for other minority and Aboriginal populations worldwide.[18,19] Differences are the result of cultural, educational, and socioeconomic factors that disparately affect minorities.

Gender

Behavior affects injuries within the first year of life. Boys are 70% more likely to die by injury than girls.[20] Differences in burn injuries follow a similar pattern; a recent systematic review shows that burns are 56% more common in males compared with females in the pediatric population worldwide.[8] Reasons for this difference are multifactorial. Studies show that boys are socialized differently than girls. They are given more independence at younger ages.[21,22] Boys have higher activity levels, engage in more risk-taking behavior, and are more impulsive than girls, increasing their risk of injury.[23]

Gender differences in burns are also observed in adults, but trends vary with burn etiology. Men are more likely to suffer electrical and chemical burns; women are affected by scald and flame injuries.[7] Burns are the only injury more common in middle-aged women compared with men.[4] In LMIC, high risk in adult females is associated with open flame and ground-level cooking, loose-fitting clothing that can easily ignite, and interpersonal violence.

AGE
Children

More than 70% of burns affect children.[24] Young children explore the world through their hands, but lack the judgment necessary to avoid hazards. Infants and children younger than 5 years are at the greatest risk.[7,25–28] Many burns are minor, but serious burns in childhood cause lifelong suffering and disability. Risk factors are related to parental education and supervision. Children of parents who have less than a high school education, are younger than 20 years old, or have 3 or more other children are at significantly greater risk.[29]

Elderly

Age-related deterioration in judgment, poor coordination and balance, and slowed responsiveness place the elderly at high risk. Older patients suffer from larger and more severe burns and have higher rates of inhalational injuries compared with younger patients.[25] Additionally, burns are poorly tolerated by seniors. Reduced physiologic capacity owing to malnutrition and medical comorbidities makes older patients more susceptible to infections, metabolic complications, and death. Many elderly patients living independently before injury are forced into nursing facilities after hospitalization.[30]

Comorbidities

Epilepsy, peripheral neuropathy, and mobility-limiting conditions, as well as cognitive disabilities are risk factors for burns. In many areas of the world, epilepsy is untreated. Burns precipitated by epileptic seizures are common throughout Africa and Asia.[31,32] If an individual falls into an open flame or onto a hot object during a seizure, bystanders are reluctant to offer help owing to traditional beliefs that the disease is contagious. Consequently, burn injuries in are often severe.[33,34] Peripheral neuropathy secondary to leprosy and diabetes is common worldwide. Scalds and contact burns owing to sensory deficits result from absence of the normal pain reflex. Neurologic and psychiatric disorders, including muscle and spinal cord conditions, dementia, and intellectual disability, affect mobility and judgment and increase risk of burn injury.

Occupation

Health and safety in the workplace are neglected in many LMIC. Regulations, when they exist, are often not enforced. Many workers are unaware of the dangers of electricity and wear little or no protective equipment.[35] The burden of upper extremity burn injuries may increase in LMIC with growing industrial development.

Regional Factors

Social habits, traditions, religious celebrations, and medicinal practices affect burn patterns. In many LMIC, open flames are used for cooking, kerosene lanterns are used for lighting, and coal embers are used for heating, all of which are common causes of burns.[36] Practices specific to particular regions put individuals at risk for unique injuries. Examples are noted.

- Steel chopsticks are popular in Korea. Hand burns occur when young children insert them into electrical sockets.[37]
- In a Southern Indian tradition, devotees rub camphor on their palms and set it on fire to enter a trance and make requests of the gods. This practice often results in full-thickness burns to the palms.[38,39]
- Lantern festivals Asian countries including China and Thailand put participants at risk for upper extremity burns. Flame burns when lighting candle wicks deeply recessed within lanterns, contact burns from holding hot

lanterns, and burns from dripping or boiling wax are all common.[40]

- Celebrations with fireworks occur throughout the world. Examples include New Year's celebrations in Europe, Fourth of July events in the United States, Greek Orthodox Easter, Jewish Purim festival, and Muslim Eid Elfitr/al-Adha feasts.[41,42] Firework-related hand burns and blast injuries often result in severe deformity or amputation.
- Crushed garlic is a pain remedy used by naturopathic providers worldwide. Garlic contains diallyl disulfide and allicin, which can cause chemical burns at the site of application or to the hands of the provider with prolonged exposure.[43]
- Cupping and coining are traditional pain relief practices in Asia and the Middle East. The ancient Greeks believed that congestion of the organs was relieved by attracting the causative pathology to the skin surface. A cup is heated with the aid of an accelerant, then placed on the affected region. Providers and patients are at risk for contact and flame burns.[44] Coining involves the application of a hot, mentholated oil. A coin is then vigorously rubbed on the affected area. Scald and friction burns often result.[45]

ACUTE BURN CARE

Much of burn morbidity can be prevented through appropriate care in the acute setting. American Burn Association guidelines mandate that hand burns be referred to a high-volume burn center for multidisciplinary, team care.[46] Although access to formal emergency medical services and certified burn centers is limited in the developing world, public education and immediate medical evaluation significantly improves prehospital and acute care.

Prehospital Care

The aims of burn first aid are to stop the burning process, cool the burn, provide pain relief, and cover the injured area. Immediate treatment decreases burn depth and improves outcome. First responders are often relatives with minimal medical knowledge. Inexperience, misconceptions, and tradition cause bystanders to provide inadequate or inappropriate care.

Appropriate first aid measures include the following.

- Ensure responder safety and prevent further injury: extinguish flames, switch off electrical current, wear gloves to protect against chemicals.
- Stop the burning process by removing clothing and copiously irrigating wounds with cool water.
- Cover the burn to provide pain relief. Dressings should be pliable, nonadherent, and impermeable. Plastic kitchen wrap is suitable, inexpensive, and widely available. Circumferential dressings should be avoided.
- Keep the patient warm.
- Seek immediate medical care.

Do not

- Apply pastes, oils, aloe, or other topical agents (aside from water) before seeking medical care
- Apply cotton dressings or any other cover that may become adherent or infected
- Apply ice directly; this may lead to further tissue damage and increase the risk of hypothermia
- Burst blisters with nonsterile needles or pins

Public education programs on burn first aid have been implemented successfully in many LMIC.[47–49] Health education in schools and communities and targeted newspaper, radio, and television campaigns increase awareness and promote the use of correct first aid measures. Low-cost interventions are possible in most countries, regardless of income level, through partnerships with the Red Cross, Red Crescent, and existing infrastructure for first aid training.

Hospital Care

Primary hospital-based treatment of a burn patient includes airway stabilization and fluid resuscitation. Estimation of burn depth and percentage of the total body surface area affected guide treatment. When intravenous access and crystalloids are available, the Parkland formula is used to estimate fluid requirements in the first 24 hours. In limited resource settings, oral rehydration therapy is routinely used and may be successful in burns up to 40% total body surface area.[50–52] Oral rehydration salts can be prepared from common ingredients (salt, sugar, baking soda, clean water) or locally available substitutes such as salted rice water or lassi, a yogurt-based drink popular in the Indian subcontinent.[53]

When possible, a thorough history should be elicited from the patient to include the mechanism of burn, the setting in which it occurred, duration of contact, and, for upper extremity burns, hand dominance, occupation, and previous injuries.

Examination of upper extremity burns focuses initially on vascular assessment, looking for weak or absent pulses, slow capillary refill, diminished sensation, and cool temperature. Circumferential burns, electrical and chemical burns, and burns involving crush injures are at high risk for vascular compromise. When vascular compromise is present or threatened, immediate escharotomy is performed. Escharotomies may be performed in the operating room or at bedside and require only a scalpel or electrocautery (**Fig. 1**). Fasciotomies are performed in cases of compartment syndrome or when pulses do not return after escharotomy.

Prevention of infection is the next priority. Burn wounds become colonized within 48 hours of injury.[54] After thorough cleansing and debridement of blisters, wounds should be dressed to minimize bacterial counts and provide a moist environment for healing. In high-resource settings, hydrocolloids, silver-impregnated gauze, and biosynthetic skin substitutes are commonplace. Topical agents such as silver sulfadiazine, aloe vera, and petroleum are effective, inexpensive alternatives. Honey, an ancient remedy for wounds, has known antimicrobial properties owing to its osmotic gradient, acidity, and inhibines.[55] Honey inhibits *Pseudomonas*, a common cause of burn wound cellulitis, and is at least as effective as silver sulfadiazine in preventing infection.[56] Banana leaves and boiled potato peel are also proven therapies. Banana leaf dressings are nonadherent owing to their waxy surface, making dressing changes less painful. Boiled potato peels are placed with the inner side down on the open wound. Both banana leaves and boiled potato peel dressings decrease wound desiccation and hasten epithelial regeneration.[57,58]

Some authors advocate enzymatic debridement with topical agents in lieu of tangential excision for partial thickness burns.[59] When available, collagenase derivatives are used. In the tropics, pastes made from pineapple, papaya, and kiwi are inexpensive alternatives.[60–62]

Deep partial and full-thickness burns require early excision and skin grafting within the first few days after injury to promote healing. A variety of instruments (ie, Weck blades and dermatomes) promote safe and effective management of burn wounds in most health care settings. Excisional debridement risks considerable blood loss; tumescent infiltration and tourniquets are useful adjuncts when blood products are limited. Early excisional debridement and grafting reduces the risk of infection and scar contractures and improves functional results. This is especially useful in upper extremity burns over joints.

REHABILITATION

Studies show that hand function is the strongest predictor of quality of life after burn in the developing world.[63] As wounds heal, restoration to pre-injury status and return to society become of primary importance. Rehabilitation begins on day 1 and includes pain management, occupational therapy, and counseling. Multidisciplinary teams of nurses, physical and occupational therapists, psychologists, and physiatrists supervise efforts in developed countries. In contrast, rehabilitation services in LMIC are rudimentary and long-term follow-up is problematic. Lack of coordinated care creates anxiety, depression, and post-traumatic stress in patients, and often leads to feelings of hopelessness—that nothing can be done to relieve suffering. Emotional withdraw is common.[64] Lack of activity and poor participation in care exacerbate secondary deformities. Fortunately, an increasing number of health care facilities worldwide are developing rehabilitation services for burn victims in both urban and rural locations.[65,66]

Uncontrolled pain is a major problem; it causes long-term psychological issues and can impede other aspects of rehabilitation. Pain management must address 3 components: (1) background pain, which is continuously present at baseline,

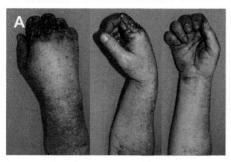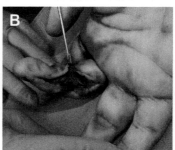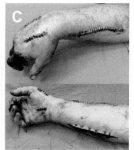

Fig. 1. High-voltage electrical burn. (*A*) Vascular compromise at presentation to emergency room. (*B*) Finger escharotomy. (*C*) Hand and forearm fasciotomies.

(2) breakthrough pain, which occurs with general movement and activities of daily living, and (3) procedural pain, which is associated with dressing changes and therapy. A combination of long- and short-acting opioids, nonsteroidal anti-inflammatory agents, acetaminophen, and gabapentin is recommended. Successful management requires ongoing evaluation of the wound burden and progress with therapy. In general, as mobility increases, pain decreases. Many burn survivors require no routine medications in the long term.[67]

Occupational therapy for upper extremity patients with burns has 2 primary goals: to maintain mobility and prevent contractures. These goals are addressed concurrently with stretching and strengthening exercises as well as pressure garments. Early active and passive range of motion and splinting should begin as soon as possible. Splints can be constructed using any available rigid materials, including plaster, Styrofoam, wood, or leather.[68] Pressure garments can be fashioned out of any elastic material. With proper instruction, patients and families can perform many of these therapies at home.

Deformity, disfigurement, and loss of independence have a profound emotional impact on burn survivors. Dependence on hand function for productivity in LMIC makes upper extremity burns particularly devastating. Psychological support and counseling are essential throughout the course of recovery. Burn survivor support groups are a low-cost solution that have been implemented in several LMIC.[69–72] Peer groups offer emotional and practical support in improving self-esteem, regaining independence, and reintegrating into the community.

POSTBURN RECONSTRUCTION

Postburn scars are inevitable. Even with the best treatment, all partial and full-thickness burns heal by scarring. Scar contractures are a common and debilitating complication in the upper extremity. Contractures occur naturally during healing to help close wounds, but have a tendency to occur over joints, compromising range of motion and overall function. The severity of a burn contracture depends on the location and depth of the burn, timing and type of initial treatment, splinting, rehabilitation, and scar care during the maturation process.[73] Contracture rates after major burns treated appropriately are as high as 39% in adults.[74–76]

Untreated, severe burns to the hands result in a characteristic posture of wrist extension, metacarpophalangeal joint hyperextension, and interphalangeal joint flexion, commonly referred to as the burn claw deformity (**Fig. 2**). This deformity results from direct thermal injury to the dorsal skin and extensor apparatus and is potentiated by immobility, edema, joint distention, and vascular compromise. In children, volar contact burns are common (**Fig. 3**).[77] Scarred or grafted skin does not grow at the same rate as the child and patients who are asymptomatic initially may develop problems over time.

Patients with symptomatic burn scar contractures present at various times after injury. Those presenting early (within months) may benefit from simple, inexpensive techniques such as compression garments, splints, and scar massage. If significant limitation in range of motion already exists, early operative intervention is advised.

Principles of upper extremity burn reconstruction include the following.

1. Excision of scarred or contracted tissue and correction of deforming forces: Burn deformities occur owing to skin injury, but over time, secondary changes occur in the muscles, ligaments, tendons, and joints. To effectively correct burn contractures, one must assess and address the contribution of each type of tissue.
2. Soft tissue coverage: Large skin defects result after burn scar contracture release. Skin grafts and flaps are frequently required to achieve wound closure (**Figs. 4 and 5**).
3. Restoration of function: Surgery on the burned upper extremity should restore shoulder abduction, elbow extension, key pinch, and power grip. The hand must have an adequate first webspace for grasp and the thumb must

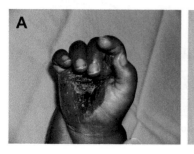
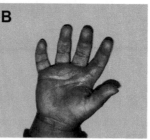

Fig. 2. Volar contact burn in child treated with dressing changes. (*A*) Five days after injury. (*B*) One month after injury.

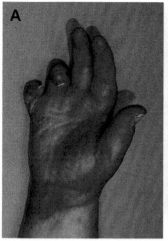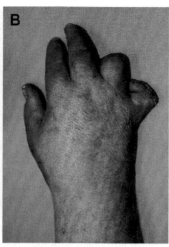

Fig. 3. (*A*) Mild burn claw deformity with metacarpal phalangeal joint hyperextension and (*B*) interphalangeal joint flexion.

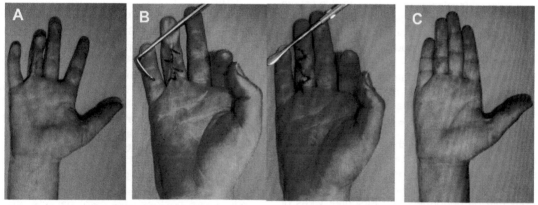

Fig. 4. Ring finger flexion contracture treated with adjacent tissue rearrangement. (*A*) Preoperative appearance. (*B*) Z-plasty design and inset. (*C*) Two months after surgery.

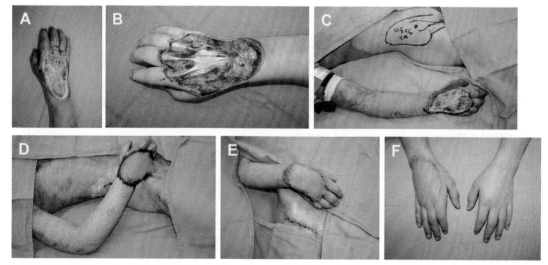

Fig. 5. Full-thickness dorsal hand burn treated with a pedicled flap. (*A*) Preoperative appearance. (*B*) After burn excision. (*C*) Groin flap design. (*D*) Flap inset. (*E*) Flap division at 4 weeks. (*F*) Seven months after surgery.

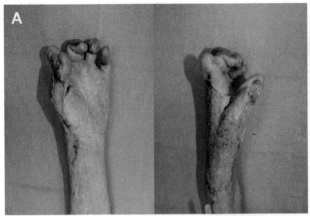
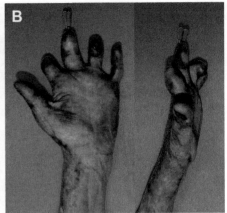

Fig. 6. Proximal interphalangeal joint fusion. (*A*) Severe hand burn resulting in flexion contracture at proximal interphalangeal joints. (*B*) Middle finger proximal interphalangeal joint fusion.

oppose adjacent fingers. Fusion of joints in a functional position is often beneficial in severe or long-standing deformities (**Fig. 6**).

4. Release proximal contractures first: Hand function is not useful without shoulder and elbow mobility.
5. Postoperative rehabilitation: Splinting, therapy, and scar control are mandatory after burn reconstruction to achieve optimal outcomes and prevent contracture recurrence.

Many reconstructive techniques are possible in resource-limited settings. Skin grafts, adjacent tissue rearrangement, and pedicled flaps (groin or abdominal) require no specialized equipment. Fusions can be performed with Kirschner wires or Steinmann pins. Splints can be constructed from available materials. Patients can perform home therapy and scar massage.

SUMMARY

Upper extremity burns are a neglected epidemic. Limited health care resources, poor infrastructure, and a lack of trained providers pose major challenges to burn treatment in the developing world. Survivors face lifelong disability with few avenues for support. Despite these obstacles, much of burn-related suffering can be prevented or minimized through education, simple interventions, and basic care. Advocacy and improved access to care are mandatory.

REFERENCES

1. World Health Organization. The global burden of disease: 2004 update. Geneva (Switzerland): World Health Organization; 2014. Available at: http://www.who.int/healthinfo/glocal_burden_disease/GBD_report_2004update_full.pdf. Accessed February 20, 2019.
2. Debas HT, Gosselin R, McCord C, et al. Surgery. In: Jamison DT, Breman JG, et al, editors. Disease control priorities in developing countries. Washington, DC: Oxford University Press; 2006.
3. Farmer PE, Kim JY. Surgery and global health: a view from beyond the OR. World J Surg 2008;32: 533–6.
4. Burns fact sheet. World Health Organization, 2018. 2019. Available at: https://www.who.int/en/newsroom/fact-sheets/detail/burns. Accessed February 16, 2019.
5. Sheridan RL, Hurley J, Smith MA, et al. The acutely burned hand: management and outcome based on a ten-year experience with 1047 acute hand burns. J Trauma 1995;38:406–11.
6. Djalalinia S, Saeedi Moghaddam S, Moradi-Lakeh M, et al. Prevalence and years lived with disability of 310 diseases and injuries in Iran and its neighboring countries, 1990-2015: findings from global burden of disease study 2015. Arch Iran Med 2017;20:392–402.
7. Marsden NJ, Battle CE, Combellack EJ, et al. The impact of socio-economic deprivation on burn injury: a nine-year retrospective study of 6441 patients. Burns 2016;42:446–52.
8. Smolle C, Cambiaso-Daniel J, Forbes AA, et al. Recent trends in burn epidemiology worldwide: a systematic review. Burns 2017;43:249–57.
9. Corlew DS, McQueen KA. International disease burden of hand burns: perspective from the global health arena. Hand Clin 2017;33:399–407.
10. Hop MJ, Polinder S, van der Vlies CH, et al. Costs of burn care: a systematic review. Wound Repair Regen 2014;22:436–50.
11. Musgrove P. Investing in health: the 1993 World Development Report of the World Bank. Bull Pan Am Health Organ 1993;27:284–6.

12. Fox-Rushby JA, Hanson K. Calculating and presenting disability adjusted life years (DALYs) in cost-effectiveness analysis. Health Policy Plan 2001;16:326–31.

13. Roberts I. Cause specific social class mortality differentials for child injury and poisoning in England and Wales. J Epidemiol Community Health 1997;51:334–5.

14. Barillo DJ, Goode R. Fire fatality study: demographics of fire victims. Burns 1996;22:85–8.

15. Istre GR, McCoy MA, Osborn L, et al. Deaths and injuries from house fires. N Engl J Med 2001;344:1911–6.

16. CDC. WISQARS nonfatal injury reports. 2017. Available at: https://webappa.cdc.gov/sasweb/ncipc/nfirates.html. Accessed February 20, 2019.

17. WISQARS fatal injury data. 2017. Available at: https://wisqars-viz.cdc.gov:8006/. Accessed February 20, 2019.

18. Duke J, Wood F, Semmens J, et al. A 26-year population-based study of burn injury hospital admissions in Western Australia. J Burn Care Res 2011;32:379–86.

19. Haik J, Liran A, Tessone A, et al. Burns in Israel: demographic, etiologic and clinical trends, 1997-2003. Isr Med Assoc J 2007;9:659–62.

20. The global burden of disease. 2004. Available at: http://www.who.int/healthinfo/global_burden_disease/GBD_report_2004update_full.pdf. Accessed February 20, 2019.

21. Block JH. Differential premises arising from differential socialization of the sexes: some conjectures. Child Dev 1983;54:1335–54.

22. Nordberg L, Rydelius PA, Zetterstrom R. Psychomotor and mental development from birth to age of four years; sex differences and their relation to home environment. Children in a new Stockholm suburb. Results from a longitudinal prospective study starting at the beginning of pregnancy. Acta Paediatr Scand Suppl 1991;378:1–25.

23. Eaton WO, Yu AP. Are sex differences in child motor activity level a function of sex differences in maturational status? Child Dev 1989;60:1005–11.

24. The global situation. 2018. Available at: http://interburns.org/about/the-global-situation/. Accessed February 20, 2019.

25. Peck MD. Epidemiology of burns throughout the world. Part I: distribution and risk factors. Burns 2011;37:1087–100.

26. Gupta M, Gupta OK, Goil P. Paediatric burns in Jaipur, India: an epidemiological study. Burns 1992;18:63–7.

27. Vilasco B, Bondurand A. Burns in Abidjan, Cote d'Ivoire. Burns 1995;21:291–6.

28. Rossi LA, Braga EC, Barruffini RC, et al. Childhood burn injuries: circumstances of occurrences and their prevention in Ribeirao Preto, Brazil. Burns 1998;24:416–9.

29. Scholer SJ, Hickson GB, Mitchel EF Jr, et al. Predictors of mortality from fires in young children. Pediatrics 1998;101:E12.

30. Alden NE, Bessey PQ, Rabbitts A, et al. Tap water scalds among seniors and the elderly: socioeconomics and implications for prevention. Burns 2007;33:666–9.

31. Courtright P, Haile D, Kohls E. The epidemiology of burns in rural Ethiopia. J Epidemiol Community Health 1993;47:19–22.

32. Fauveau V, Blanchet T. Deaths from injuries and induced abortion among rural Bangladeshi women. Social Sci Med 1989;29:1121–7.

33. Al-Qattan MM. Burns in epileptics in Saudi Arabia. Burns 2000;26:561–3.

34. Al-Qattan MM, Al-Zahrani K. A review of burns related to traditions, social habits, religious activities, festivals and traditional medical practices. Burns 2009;35:476–81.

35. Choong M, Chy D, Guevarra JR, et al. Clinical management of electrical burns in the developing world: a case of electrical burn injury left untreated leading to amputation. BMJ Case Rep 2017;2017 [pii:bcr2016218188].

36. Patel A, Sawh-Martinez RF, Sinha I, et al. Establishing sustainable international burn missions: lessons from India. Ann Plast Surg 2013;71:31–3.

37. Lee JW, Jang YC, Oh SJ. Paediatric electrical burn: outlet injury caused by steel chopstick misuse. Burns 2004;30:244–7.

38. Tay YG, Tan KK. Unusual ritual burns of the hand. Burns 1996;22:409–12.

39. Lewis DM, Balakrishnan S, Coady MS, et al. Camphor burns to the palm: an unusual self-inflicted burn. Burns 2007;33:672.

40. Chan ES, Chan EC, Ho WS, et al. Boiling wax burn in mid-autumn festival in Hong Kong. Burns 1997;23:629–30.

41. Vassilia K, Eleni P, Dimitrios T. Firework-related childhood injuries in Greece: a national problem. Burns 2004;30:151–3.

42. Zohar Z, Waksman I, Stolero J, et al. [Injury from fireworks and firecrackers during holidays]. Harefuah 2004;143:698–701, 68.

43. Al-Qattan MM. Garlic burns: case reports with an emphasis on associated and underlying pathology. Burns 2009;35:300–2.

44. Kose AA, Karabagli Y, Cetin C. An unusual cause of burns due to cupping: complication of a folk medicine remedy. Burns 2006;32:126–7.

45. Amshel CE, Caruso DM. Vietnamese "coining": a burn case report and literature review. J Burn Care Rehabil 2000;21:112–4.

46. Guidelines for the operation of burn centers. 2019. Available at: http://ameriburn.org/wp-content/uploads/2017/05/burncenterreferralcriteria.pdf. Accessed February 23, 2019.

47. Ghosh A, Bharat R. Domestic burns prevention and first aid awareness in and around Jamshedpur, India: strategies and impact. Burns 2000;26:605–8.

48. Husum H, Gilbert M, Wisborg T, et al. Rural prehospital trauma systems improve trauma outcome in low-income countries: a prospective study from North Iraq and Cambodia. J Trauma 2003;54:1188–96.

49. King L, Thomas M, Gatenby K, et al. "First aid for scalds" campaign: reaching Sydney's Chinese, Vietnamese, and Arabic speaking communities. Inj Prev 1999;5:104–8.

50. Vyas KS, Wong LK. Oral rehydration solutions for burn management in the field and underdeveloped regions: a review. Int J Burns Trauma 2013;3:130–6.

51. Michell MW, Oliveira HM, Kinsky MP, et al. Enteral resuscitation of burn shock using World Health Organization oral rehydration solution: a potential solution for mass casualty care. J Burn Care Res 2006;27:819–25.

52. Kramer GC, Michell MW, Oliveira H, et al. Oral and enteral resuscitation of burn shock the historical record and implications for mass casualty care. Eplasty 2010;10 [pii:e56].

53. Jeng J, Gibran N, Peck M. Burn care in disaster and other austere settings. Surg Clin North America 2014;94:893–907.

54. Church D, Elsayed S, Reid O, et al. Burn wound infections. Clin Microbiol Rev 2006;19:403–34.

55. Israili ZH. Antimicrobial properties of honey. Am J Ther 2014;21:304–23.

56. Subrahmanyam M. A prospective randomised clinical and histological study of superficial burn wound healing with honey and silver sulfadiazine. Burns 1998;24:157–61.

57. Guenova E, Hoetzenecker W, Kisuze G, et al. Banana leaves as an alternative wound dressing. Dermatol Surg 2013;39:290–7.

58. Keswani MH, Vartak AM, Patil A, et al. Histological and bacteriological studies of burn wounds treated with boiled potato peel dressings. Burns 1990;16:137–43.

59. Cordts T, Horter J, Vogelpohl J, et al. Enzymatic debridement for the treatment of severely burned upper extremities - early single center experiences. BMC Dermatol 2016;16:8.

60. Starley IF, Mohammed P, Schneider G, et al. The treatment of paediatric burns using topical papaya. Burns 1999;25:636–9.

61. Atiyeh B, Masellis A, Conte C. Optimizing burn treatment in developing low-and middle-income countries with limited health care resources (Part 2). Ann Burns Fire Disasters 2009;22:189–95.

62. Mohajeri G, Masoudpour H, Heidarpour M, et al. The effect of dressing with fresh kiwifruit on burn wound healing. Surgery 2010;148:963–8.

63. McMahon HA, Ndem I, Gampper L, et al. Quantifying burn injury-related disability and quality of life in the developing world: a primer for patient-centered resource allocation. Ann Plast Surg 2019;82(6S Suppl 5):S433–6.

64. Wallis H, Renneberg B, Ripper S, et al. Emotional distress and psychosocial resources in patients recovering from severe burn injury. J Burn Care Res 2006;27:734–41.

65. Karunadasa KP, Perera C, Kanagaratnum V, et al. Burns due to acid assaults in Sri Lanka. J Burn Care Res 2010;31:781–5.

66. Mathangi Ramakrishnan K, Jayaraman V, Andal A, et al. Paediatric rehabilitation in a developing country–India in relation to aetiology, consequences and outcome in a group of 459 burnt children. Pediatr Rehabil 2004;7:145–9.

67. Young A. Rehabilitation of burn injuries. Phys Med Rehabil Clin N Am 2002;13:85–108, vi.

68. Thomforde DW. A technique for making hand splints from Styrofoam and plywood. Asia Pacific Disability Rehabilitation Journal 2005;16:93–101.

69. Teixeira Nicolosi J, Fernandes de Carvalho V, Llonch Sabates A. A quantitative, cross-sectional study of depression and self-esteem in teenage and young adult burn victims in rehabilitation. Ostomy Wound Manage 2013;59:22–9.

70. Kornhaber R, Wilson A, Abu-Qamar M, et al. Inpatient peer support for adult burn survivors-a valuable resource: a phenomenological analysis of the Australian experience. Burns 2015;41:110–7.

71. Jagnoor J, Lukaszyk C, Fraser S, et al. Rehabilitation practices for burn survivors in low and middle income countries: a literature review. Burns 2018;44:1052–64.

72. Gouthi SC. A impact of supportive psychotherapy on burn patients. Indian J Burns 2011;19:10–5.

73. Gupta RK, Jindal N, Kamboj K. Neglected post burns contracture of hand in children: analysis of contributory socio-cultural factors and the impact of neglect on outcome. J Clin Orthop Trauma 2014;5:215–20.

74. Chapman TT. Burn scar and contracture management. J Trauma 2007;62:S8.

75. Klein MB, Lezotte DL, Fauerbach JA, et al. The National Institute on Disability and Rehabilitation Research burn model system database: a tool for the multicenter study of the outcome of burn injury. J Burn Care Res 2007;28:84–96.

76. Schwarz RJ. Management of postburn contractures of the upper extremity. J Burn Care Res 2007;28:212–9.

77. Brown M, Coffee T, Adenuga P, et al. Outcomes of outpatient management of pediatric burns. J Burn Care Res 2014;35:388–94.

Treating Pediatric Hand Problems in a Low-resource Environment

Michelle A. James, MD*

KEYWORDS

- Pediatric hand surgery • Congenital hand anomalies • Low-resource environment • Global health

KEY POINTS

- Hand anomalies, injuries, and neuromuscular diseases affect children's hand function, especially in low-resource environments where prevention and early treatment are not readily available.
- Surgical care is the most important global health need of the next decade, and short-term pediatric hand surgeon trips to resource-poor countries are part of the strategy to meet this need.
- Pediatric hand surgery can improve lifelong function with few risks, although children with hand anomalies may have associated conditions that increase their risk from anesthesia.
- Children with neuromuscular conditions can benefit from carefully planned hand and upper limb surgery, as can children with postburn and posttraumatic deformities.
- It is deeply gratifying for surgeons to use their highly developed skills to benefit children who would otherwise not receive treatment.

INTRODUCTION

Children's hand function is affected by many different conditions, including congenital malformations and deformities, neuromuscular disease, trauma (including burns), and posttraumatic deformities. Although many of these individual conditions are uncommon or rare, their combined burden is considerable, especially in low-resource environments where prevention and early treatment may not be readily available.[1,2]

Surgical care is the most important global health need of the next decade.[3] Well-trained surgeons from high-income countries have responded to this need by using their skills to care for people with surgical problems in low-resource environments, and to impart knowledge and skills to local surgeons.[4,5] Although the surgical care and training provided by short-term surgeon trips

may not be sufficient to achieve sustained improvements in care,[6] as part of a strategy that includes training health care professionals and providing access to resources (equipment and supplies), it is an important component of the road map to better global surgical care.[7–10]

Hand problems are especially amenable to the short-term service trip approach, for several reasons. Hand conditions can be disabling, and are often treatable with low-risk, low-resource surgery; furthermore, local subspecialty care is often not available in resource-limited environments.[11] Treatment of pediatric hand problems is especially compelling, because growth may adversely affect outcomes, and resulting disability is lifelong.

This article addresses important considerations for providing effective care of pediatric hand conditions in low-resource environments, and

Disclosure: The author has no financial relationship with a commercial company that has a direct financial interest in subject matter or materials discussed in the article. She is Deputy Editor of Hand and Upper Extremity for the *Journal of Bone and Joint Surgery*.
Shriners Hospital for Children Northern California, University of California Davis School of Medicine, 2425 Stockton Boulevard, Sacramento, CA 95817, USA
* Shriners Hospital for Children, Northern California 2425 Stockton Boulevard, Sacramento, CA 95817.
E-mail address: mjames@shrinenet.org

Hand Clin 35 (2019) 467–478
https://doi.org/10.1016/j.hcl.2019.07.011

shares guidelines for approaches to treating specific pediatric hand and upper limb conditions.

CONSIDERATIONS FOR TREATING PEDIATRIC HAND PROBLEMS IN RESOURCE-POOR ENVIRONMENTS

The process necessary to match a pediatric hand surgeon's skills with the patients' needs varies with the environment and many other factors, but general considerations apply to guide the planning and execution of short-term service trips[7,12–16] (**Box 1**).

Personal Motivations and Goals

A thoughtful inventory by surgeons of their motivations and goals will inform and influence trip selection and planning. In addition to other personal reasons, pediatric hand surgeons are motivated by a desire to use their specialized skills to help children and teach local surgeons and trainees. Their goals include accomplishing this successfully in the context of a different culture and health care system. The desire to help is necessary, but not sufficient, to facilitate a fulfilling short-term service trip.

Although all surgeons are likely to learn new skills on service trips, those with extensive experience will be more comfortable in a resource-poor environment. Experience informs successful patient selection, because experienced surgeons who know their limits are more likely to select cases that will have good outcomes; it also helps intraoperatively, when unexpected events occur (eg, instruments and equipment break or are unavailable), because

---

Box 1
Considerations for treating pediatric hand problems in resource-poor environments

Personal motivation and goals of the surgeon

Communication, cultural competency, local history, and current events

Planning in collaboration with hosts

Team composition

Travel and health tips and safety measures

Patient selection and operating room schedule

Preoperative preparation

Surgery

Postoperative plan

End-of-trip debriefing

Sustainability

---

the more experienced surgeons know alternative ways to accomplish a surgical goal. Less experienced surgeons planning a service trip would be wise to partner with a veteran, because most surgeons feel out of their comfort zone on their early trips, and can benefit from reassurance that this is a normal response to a challenging situation.

Hand surgeons tend to be meticulous individuals with high performance standards. These personality traits help them take good care of patients. Adjusting to suboptimal circumstances can be disconcerting and frustrating. Surgeons who thrive in resource-poor environments manage to adapt to difficult and unexpected situations while maintaining attention to important details.

Communication, Cultural Competency, Local History, and Current Events

In many resource-limited countries, English is not the native language. Host surgeons and residents may speak English, but this varies, and is less likely among staff at public hospitals, where pediatric hand surgeons are more likely to work. Accurate communication is critically important during trip planning, execution, and follow-up. The best way to communicate is in the host's language. If the pediatric hand surgeon is not able to speak and understand the local language fluently, a translator will be necessary, and the surgeon should learn a few key phrases in the local language that communicate a warm greeting and appreciation.

Before the trip, the pediatric hand surgeon should seek to understand the local culture. Interactions such as gestures, shaking hands, and eye contact may have different connotations than in the United States. Surgeons should also pursue knowledge of local history and current events, particularly the type of government, the names of leaders, and the impact of former actions of the United States on the country (this is particularly appropriate for Mexico and Central American countries), before their trips. For hosts and local citizens, their history provides context for the surgeon's visit, and when the surgeon attempts to understand their perspective, it facilitates communication and goodwill.

It is much easier throughout the trip to interact primarily with US team members, but attempts to interact with local hosts, even if they seem difficult and awkward, are appreciated and help develop richer and more durable relationships. It is especially important to avoid caucusing with team members in English in the presence of non–English-speaking hosts.

Trip Planning in Collaboration with Hosts

Planning a trip in collaboration with a supportive organization such as Health Volunteers Overseas (https://hvousa.org/), or The Touching Hands Project[17] (http://www.assh.org/touching-hands), facilitates this process and is highly recommended. If a pediatric hand surgery team has not previously visited the planned location, and is not working with a supportive organization, the first step is an assessment visit, including a survey of local needs, qualifications of local personnel, operating room and anesthesia equipment, supplies, availability of therapists, and other factors such as accommodation and transportation for the team. Planning a service trip to a new location can be time consuming and complex; several recent publications are available for guidance.[7,10,15,18]

Regardless of the involvement of a supportive organization or previous trips, local hosts are planning partners, especially with respect to trip timing (eg, avoiding local holidays, when elective operating room time and staff may not be available), team composition, and packing (equipment and supplies that are not available locally). The team should bring sufficient operating room attire for team members to use throughout the trip (scrubs, hats, masks, shoe covers, gloves) to avoid depleting the local stock. Scrubs and any leftover attire can be donated to the local hospital at the end of the trip. The team should also consider bringing thumb drives loaded with pediatric hand resources (eg, articles, books) to give to local hosts and trainees; pens, pins, and other swag items from their home hospital for staff; and a generous supply of small safe toys to give to patients.

Local hosts should prescreen and refer children with hand problems to the team's clinic, based on the hosts' and teams' competencies and local need. If possible, a survey of local needs is helpful,[19] but this information is difficult to acquire in advance.

Team Composition

The team must include at least 1 experienced pediatric hand surgeon. Resource-limited environments are not suitable for learning pediatric hand techniques, or trying new operations; it is sufficiently daunting to operate with different (and frequently inadequate) equipment and inexperienced assistants who speak a different language. The most important role of the experienced surgeon is patient selection (discussed later).

Other team members include a second pediatric hand surgeon (in case one becomes ill, or 2 operating rooms become available) and a pediatric occupational therapist (who can teach pediatric hand function assessment techniques, splint fabrication, and postoperative therapy protocols to local rehabilitation staff). Residents or hand fellows may also be included (their role is to assist and learn how to select patients and develop relationships with local hosts, because it is not appropriate to use patients in low-resource settings to provide added experience for trainees) along with additional volunteers, including nurse practitioners or physician assistants, and premedical and medical students. At least 1 team member should be fluent in the local language, in order to serve as translator. Roles for each team member should be defined in advance, including team leader, record keeper, photographer, and toy distributors (discussed later). The team may also include operating room nurses and technicians and an anesthesiologist; the need for these skill sets can be determined by the trip planning assessment. In general, for sustainability and to support local skill acquisition, it is preferable to use local staff as much as possible; fortunately, this approach is suitable for pediatric hand surgery, which is inherently less risky than cleft palate or spine surgery (a major exception to this is the risk associated with operating on children with syndromes; discussed later). Of course, the team also includes the local hosts, usually a chief of service (orthopedics or plastic surgery); a local staff-level surgeon who will be responsible for assisting with scheduling, equipment, surgery, rounding on patients, and follow-up; and local orthopedic or plastic surgery residents (**Fig. 1**).

Several months before the trip, all clinician members of the team should submit any documents required by the local hospital and health ministry, including licenses, diplomas, and so forth, and the trip leader should carry copies of all documents. In addition, several weeks before the trip, the team leader should submit lists of all supplies and equipment they plan to transport in their luggage to the local health ministry and customs department, as required, and pack a copy of the list in each piece of luggage. Supportive organizations are familiar with local regulations and can assist with these measures, which helps the team avoid denial of privileges by the local hospital, and confiscation of equipment and supplies.

Travel and Health Tips and Safety Measures

The team members should familiarize themselves with recommended vaccinations and medications to carry with them, in addition to insect repellant, which is important to avoid bites from mosquitoes

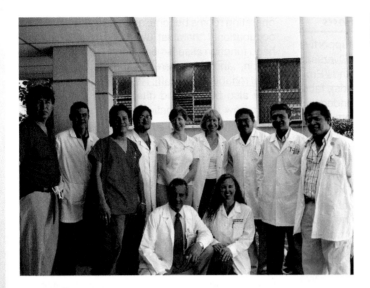

Fig. 1. Nicaraguan and US pediatric hand surgery team, Hospital Fernando Velez Paiz, Managua, Nicaragua.

carrying malaria, dengue, or chikungunya viruses (**Fig. 2**). Young women traveling to areas where the Zika virus is endemic should be aware that fetal exposure to this virus causes microcephaly. The Centers for Disease Control and Prevention Web site (https://www.cdc.gov) and the US State Department Web site (https://travel.state.gov/) include up-to-date information about travel, by country. In addition, the State Department sponsors a travel enrollment program (https://step.state.gov/STEP/); enrolled travelers are notified of any unexpected situations in the country in which they are traveling.

Patient Selection

Typically, local hosts screen children with hand problems and refer them to a clinic, held the first day of the trip (**Fig. 3**). The team members designated as recorders keep a list of patients seen, including age, diagnosis, and recommended treatment, from which a list of operative candidates is compiled. On the first trip to a new location, simple cases should be posted first, so the team can gauge the capabilities of the operating room and anesthesia staff. Cases that require more intense follow-up should also be posted early in the trip.

All patients must be evaluated for comorbidities, especially illnesses or deformities that affect the airway or otherwise increase the risk of anesthesia (discussed later). One of the benefits of creating a sustainable rotation at a local hospital (discussed later) is that, for pediatric hand conditions that require staging, surgery later in childhood, or special equipment that

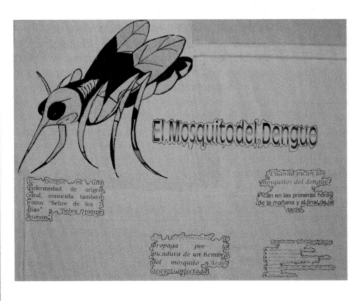

Fig. 2. Dengue fever poster, Hospital Fernando Velez Paiz, Managua, Nicaragua.

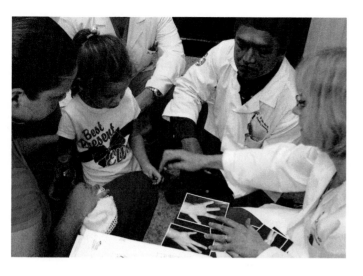

Fig. 3. Pediatric clinic, planning an index pollicization. Hospital Fernando Velez Paiz, Managua, Nicaragua.

is not currently available, the child can return for future care. This benefit relieves pressure on the surgeon to perform suboptimally compatible procedures, or to operate at a suboptimal age or without proper equipment. In addition, infants should be examined for occult treatable orthopedic comorbidities, such as developmental dislocation of the hip and torticollis, so that treatment can be initiated.

Surgeons should not be reluctant to make the difficult decision to decline to operate. This decision may be made for ethical reasons (eg, the risk-benefit ratio is not in the patient's favor) or practical reasons (eg, the surgeon does not have the skill set or equipment to perform the operation needed). The surgeon may also need to resist the local surgeons' enthusiasm for observing a technically complex procedure. The same age guidelines for surgery that are used at the surgeon's home institution in order to diminish risks of anesthesia, including neurotoxicity, should be used at the host institution.[20] The surgeon should respect local preoperative testing and criteria for safe anesthesia. It is much better to forego surgery than to cause a complication that might be difficult or impossible to treat locally. First, do no harm.

The team member designated as photographer takes photographs of all cases planned for surgery after asking for permission from the parents. The toy distributors provide each patient with a toy.

Preoperative Preparation

Accurate and comprehensive communication with the patients' parents is critically important, and is especially difficult because it occurs during the chaos of clinic day. Communication with the local surgeons and anesthesiologists is equally important. The entire team should hold a preoperative planning meeting at the end of clinic day to review the surgical schedule for the entire trip, and should also meet at the end of each day thereafter to discuss the schedule and equipment and supplies needed for the next day. Sterilization of implants, including Kirschner wires, may need to be planned 24 hours in advance.

The visiting surgeons should model adherence to the World Health Organization (WHO) Surgical Safety Checklist[21,22] (**Fig. 4**) and, if the local hospital is not using this, take the opportunity to educate key personnel, especially the chiefs of surgery and anesthesia and the operating room manager about the use of this checklist.

Before each procedure, in addition to checking the elements of the WHO checklist, the designated team members should assemble suture and dressings.

Surgery

With the help of the local surgeons, pediatric hand surgeons should double-check the availability of equipment and supplies. Intraoperative communication is especially difficult, and misunderstandings are common.

Pediatric hand surgeons should endeavor to teach surgical technique to the designated local staff surgeons and local residents, at levels commensurate with their abilities (**Fig. 5**). Visiting trainees may remain unscrubbed, to take photographs and assist with acquiring and opening supplies and equipment.

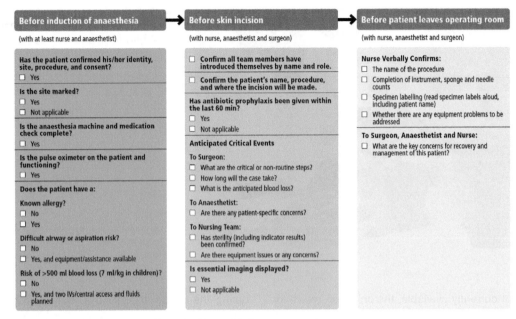

Before induction of anaesthesia	Before skin incision	Before patient leaves operating room
(with at least nurse and anaesthetist)	(with nurse, anaesthetist and surgeon)	(with nurse, anaesthetist and surgeon)

Before induction of anaesthesia
(with at least nurse and anaesthetist)

Has the patient confirmed his/her identity, site, procedure, and consent?
☐ Yes

Is the site marked?
☐ Yes
☐ Not applicable

Is the anaesthesia machine and medication check complete?
☐ Yes

Is the pulse oximeter on the patient and functioning?
☐ Yes

Does the patient have a:

Known allergy?
☐ No
☐ Yes

Difficult airway or aspiration risk?
☐ No
☐ Yes, and equipment/assistance available

Risk of >500 ml blood loss (7 ml/kg in children)?
☐ No
☐ Yes, and two IVs/central access and fluids planned

Before skin incision
(with nurse, anaesthetist and surgeon)

☐ **Confirm all team members have introduced themselves by name and role.**

☐ **Confirm the patient's name, procedure, and where the incision will be made.**

Has antibiotic prophylaxis been given within the last 60 min?
☐ Yes
☐ Not applicable

Anticipated Critical Events

To Surgeon:
☐ What are the critical or non-routine steps?
☐ How long will the case take?
☐ What is the anticipated blood loss?

To Anaesthetist:
☐ Are there any patient-specific concerns?

To Nursing Team:
☐ Has sterility (including indicator results) been confirmed?
☐ Are there equipment issues or any concerns?

Is essential imaging displayed?
☐ Yes
☐ Not applicable

Before patient leaves operating room
(with nurse, anaesthetist and surgeon)

Nurse Verbally Confirms:
☐ The name of the procedure
☐ Completion of instrument, sponge and needle counts
☐ Specimen labelling (read specimen labels aloud, including patient name)
☐ Whether there are any equipment problems to be addressed

To Surgeon, Anaesthetist and Nurse:
☐ What are the key concerns for recovery and management of this patient?

This checklist is not intended to be comprehensive. Additions and modifications to fit local practice are encouraged.

Fig. 4. WHO surgical safety checklist. (*Courtesy of* World Health Organization. WHO Surgical Checklist. Available at: https://www.who.int/patientsafety/topics/safe-surgery/checklist/en/.)

Postoperative Planning, Future Planning, and Sustainability

Postoperatively, in addition to providing a detailed plan for postoperative care, the team should hold a debriefing meeting to discuss which elements of the case went well, and which could be improved.

At the end of the trip, the entire team should meet (preferably over a delicious local meal) to debrief, evaluate goals, and plan future trips based on local needs.

Sustainability depends on many factors, only some of which are under the control of the visiting surgeons. Surgeons can commit to midterm services, and focus on providing development and education for local surgeons[9,23,24] and local needs assessments,[19] including promoting local surgeons for surgeon scholar programs (https://posna.org/Physician-Education/COUR). Ideally,

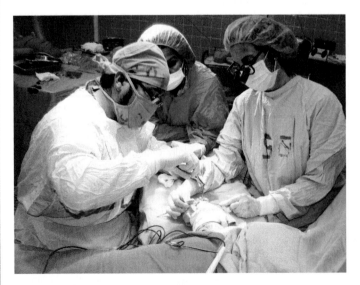

Fig. 5. US pediatric hand surgeon teaching a Nicaraguan resident. Hospital Fernando Velez Paiz, Managua, Nicaragua.

visiting surgeons will not duplicate or undermine local capacity, and will not create dependency on foreign free care.

APPROACHES TO TREATING SPECIFIC PEDIATRIC HAND AND UPPER EXTREMITY CONDITIONS
Congenital Malformations and Deformities

Congenital malformations and deformities are among the most common hand conditions seen on pediatric hand service trips in low-resource environments.[23] The pediatric hand surgeon should examine the entire child, remembering that syndromes associated with hand malformations may have occult manifestations, and that some of these make general anesthesia riskier.

Congenital differences that are not usually associated with increased risk of anesthesia

Every patient should be carefully examined for comorbidities that can increase the risk of anesthesia, especially cardiac or airway issues. The conditions discussed here are not usually associated with increased anesthetic risk, and their surgical treatment is straightforward.

Polydactyly and syndactyly can be treated by standard techniques (**Fig. 6**). Parents should be informed that these conditions may be inheritable.

The bands and acrosyndactyly that characterize constriction band syndrome can be treated by standard techniques, including syndactyly release and web-space deepening. This condition is frequently bilateral. Toe syndactylies do not require treatment. Free vascularized toe transfer may be indicated for older children with both thumbs missing, however, this should only be attempted by surgeons experienced in this technique, at a center with appropriate support.

Unilateral malformations such as transverse failure of formation and symbrachydactyly are unlikely to substantially affect function,[25,26] so reconstruction of the affected hand is either not necessary (failure of formation) or can remain simple (release of syndactylies, deepening of web spaces). Children with symbrachydactyly should be checked for Poland syndrome, primarily for the purpose of anticipatory guidance of the parents. Free vascularized toe transfers are not indicated when 1 hand is normal.

For children with cleft hands, reconstruction of prehension takes precedence over closing clefts, and, if the cleft is the only space capable of prehension, closure is contraindicated. Reconstruction of cleft feet is not usually necessary. The syndactyly and thumb hypoplasia that accompany ulnar deficiency may be treated with standard techniques. Macrodactyly may be treated with ray resection (**Fig. 7**), or debulking and/or epiphyseodesis as indicated.

Proximal radioulnar synostosis may be treated with rotational osteotomies if the hand is hyperpronated and this interferes with function. Internal fixation may not be available in resource-limited conditions, so an alternative technique that does not require internal fixation (as described by Ezaki and Oishi[27]) may be helpful.

Congenital differences that are likely to be associated with increased anesthetic risk

Pediatric hand surgeons can frequently improve function for children with arthrogryposis multiplex congenital (AMC) and distal arthrogryposis syndromes.[28] For children with AMC, posterior elbow capsulotomy and triceps lengthening improve passive elbow flexion,[29] dorsal carpal wedge osteotomy improves wrist extension,[30] and index dorsal rotation flap improves thumb abduction.[31] Children with distal arthrogryposis can benefit from index dorsal rotation flap and (for older children) thumb metacarpophalangeal

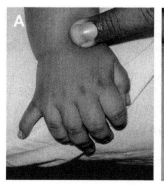
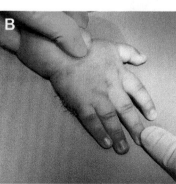

Fig. 6. (*A*) Postaxial polydactyly (preoperative). (*B*) Postaxial polydactyly (postoperative).

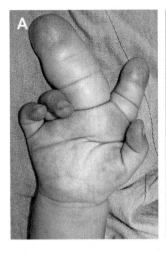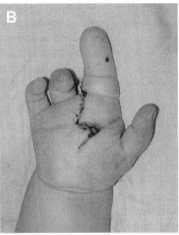

Fig. 7. (*A*) Macrodactyly (preoperative). (*B*) Macrodactyly, after long finger ray resection.

arthrodesis. However, children with both types of arthrogryposis have airway challenges, and intravenous access may be difficult. Surgeons should forego operating on children with arthrogryposis unless they are confident that the anesthesiologist has experience treating children with these conditions.

Radial longitudinal deficiency and thumb deficiency (**Fig. 8**) are associated with several different syndromes, many of which preclude safe anesthesia. Children with these conditions should be carefully examined for airway anomalies, cardiac conditions, and thrombocytopenia. Centralization requires long-term splinting, which may not be

available in a resource-poor environment. Index pollicization is one of the most helpful operations a pediatric surgeon can perform, but, like all operations in resource-limited environments, should be undertaken only if the surgeon has experience performing this operation.

Dysplasias

Dysplastic conditions require a pediatric orthopedic approach, because their treatment may vary with age and may include growth modulation procedures. Hereditary multiple osteochondromatosis is followed throughout childhood; osteochondromas are removed if they interfere with motion or cause pain, or if they are bothersome at the end of growth. Children with this condition should be examined for symptoms of myelopathy from intraspinal osteochondromas,[32] although MRI and spine surgery may not be available in resource-poor environments. The enchondromas of Ollier disease do not usually require surgical treatment until near the end of growth, when debulking and bone grafting may be helpful.[33] Long-term follow-up is an important component of treatment of these conditions.

Neuromuscular Conditions

In general, children with neuromuscular conditions such as brachial plexus birth injury (BPBI) and cerebral palsy require therapy, special surgical expertise, and long-term follow-up. Pediatric hand surgeons may find opportunities for surgical treatment in specific circumstances.

Brachial plexus birth injury

Ideally, infants with BPBI are examined serially starting soon after birth, to map the trajectory of their recovery. Those who do not recover active

Fig. 8. A 3-year-old child with bilateral thumb deficiency and right radius deficiency.

elbow flexion against gravity by 6 months of age are treated with nerve surgery.[34] Pediatric hand surgeons may wish to consider brachial plexus exploration and grafting (if they have expertise in this technique), but nerve transfers to restore elbow flexion and shoulder abduction are likely safer and possibly just as effective.[35] Shoulder subluxation may occur in infancy; it is usually diagnosed by ultrasonography[36] and treated with botulinum toxin injections[37] or arthroscopic release and tendon transfer.[38] Ultrasonography, botulinum toxin, and arthroscopy are not likely to be available in a low-resource environment. When passive external rotation of the shoulder in adduction is less than 60°, the shoulder is likely subluxated[36]; pediatric hand surgeons experienced in care of infants with BPBI should consider open release of the subscapularis at its insertion or origin, with or without tendon transfers, depending on the child's age and other factors.

Older children with BPBI can be treated according to standard indications for shoulder external rotation tendon transfers,[39] humeral rotational osteotomies (if fixation is available),[40] biceps rerouting,[41] and forearm derotational osteotomy.[27]

Upper extremity cerebral palsy
Treatment of upper extremity cerebral palsy is a complex endeavor and may be further complicated because the underlying causes of cerebral palsy may differ in low-resource environments, causing spasticity patterns unfamiliar to pediatric hand surgeons. However, carefully planned surgery can improve function for children with this condition.[42]

The surgeon should observe whether the child uses the affected extremity during simple bimanual activities, and, if so, the position of the elbow, forearm, wrist, and thumb. The surgeon should also assess isolated muscle control (extensor pollicis longus, for rerouting) and the phasic activity of a muscle during grasp and release (flexor carpi ulnaris, for wrist extension transfer), and follow the usual indications for common operations (biceps and brachialis release, pronator teres release, wrist extension transfer and extensor pollicis longus rerouting, adductor pollicis release).[43] Postoperatively, the hand surgery team should provide postoperative protocols for the local team.

For adolescents with wrist flexion contracture, proximal row carpectomy and wrist arthrodesis is helpful,[44] if internal fixation is available. Surgeons may need to combine this operation with fractional lengthening of the finger flexors. Thumb flexion contracture can be simultaneously treated with metacarpophalangeal joint arthrodesis.

Postburn and Posttraumatic Deformities

Pediatric hand teams may encounter patients with acute hand burns and trauma; the treatment of

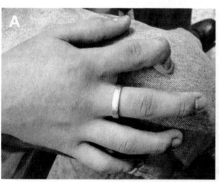
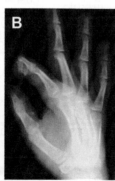
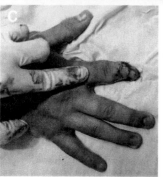

Fig. 9. (*A*) Index finger deformity 10 years after an electrical burn. (*B*) Radiograph of the same index finger. (*C*) The same index finger following distal interphalangeal joint arthrodesis.

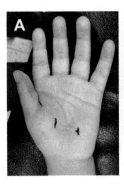
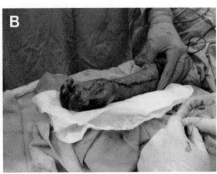

Fig. 10. (*A*) A 5-year-old 1 year following a fall on a sharp rock that lacerated all 9 flexor tendons (zone 3) and the median nerve. (*B*) The same patient following nerve and tendon grafts.

these is beyond the scope of this article. Surgeons should follow the general principles of keeping the treatment simple and within the capacity of the local host institution.

Postburn contractures and posttrauma deformities are common in low-resource environments. Fixation of nonunions may be challenging, because internal fixation options are often limited. Finger, wrist, elbow, and axillary contractures can be released according to standard indications, and defects covered with full-thickness or split-thickness skin graft, with substantial improvement in function.[45] Osteotomies may be necessary for long-standing contractures, and arthrodesis of interphalangeal joints may be indicated (**Fig. 9**). Old nerve and tendon damage is also commonly seen. Nerve and tendon grafts can be successfully performed (**Fig. 10**), if necessary in a staged fashion. The surgical team may wish to bring Hunter rods for reconstruction of old flexor tendon injuries, as long as they are planning to return to complete this staged procedure.

Research

Partnering with the host surgeons to investigate questions that are important to them can be very rewarding.[12,19,23] Before initiating any research involving patients, the research team should follow all local human subjects regulations, in addition to obtaining permission from the visiting surgeons' host institution human subjects committee. A sustainable local program is required, and a translator who is familiar with the local culture is necessary to obtain informed consent.

SUMMARY

It is deeply gratifying for surgeons to use their highly developed skills to benefit people who would otherwise not receive treatment (**Fig. 11**). To do so effectively requires communication, planning, teamwork, cultural sensitivity, and adaptability. Las características nicaragüenses (Nicaraguan personality traits) include la paciencia, el ojo de un águila, y buen humor; these are also desirable characteristics for surgeons traveling to resource-poor environments. The rewards of such travel (personal growth, expanded surgical skills, grateful patients and parents, new colleagues) are immeasurable.

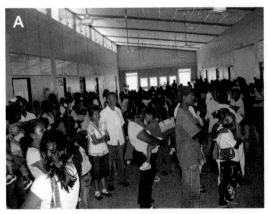
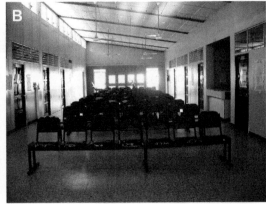

Fig. 11. (*A*) Waiting room for pediatric hand clinic (at the beginning of clinic), Hospital Velez Paiz, Managua, Nicaragua. (*B*) Waiting room after pediatric hand clinic, Hospital Velez Paiz, Managua, Nicaragua.

REFERENCES

1. Awe OO, Oladele OA, Olabanji JK, et al. Epidemiology of hand injuries seen at two teaching hospitals in Southern Nigeria. East Cent Afr J Surg 2015;20(2): 44–8.
2. Chung KY, Hanemaayer A, Poenaru D. Pediatric hand surgery in global health: the role for international outreach. Ann Plast Surg 2017;78(2):162–70.
3. Global Surgery. The essentials. New York: Springer Science+Business Media; 2017.
4. Casey KM. The global impact of surgical volunteerism. Surg Clin North Am 2007;87(4):949–60.
5. Chung KC, Kotsis SV. Teaching pediatric hand surgery in Vietnam. Hand (N Y) 2007;2(1):16–24.
6. Isaacson G, Drum ET, Cohen MS. Surgical missions to developing countries: ethical conflicts. Otolaryngol Head Neck Surg 2010;143(4):476–9.
7. Butler M, Drum E, Evans FM, et al. Guidelines and checklists for short-term missions in global pediatric surgery: recommendations from the American Academy of Pediatrics Delivery of Surgical Care Global Health Subcommittee, American Pediatric Surgical Association. Paediatr Anaesth 2018;28(5): 392–410.
8. Ng-Kamstra JS, Greenberg SLM, Abdullah F, et al. Global surgery 2030: a roadmap for high income country actors. BMJ Glob Health 2016;1(1):e000011.
9. Shrime MG, Sleemi A, Ravilla TD. Charitable platforms in global surgery: a systematic review of their effectiveness, cost-effectiveness, sustainability, and role training. World J Surg 2015;39(1):10–20.
10. Schneider WJ, Politis GD, Gosain AK, et al. Volunteers in plastic surgery guidelines for providing surgical care for children in the less developed world. Plast Reconstr Surg 2011;127(6):2477–86.
11. Chung KC. Volunteering in the developing world: The 2003–2004 Sterling Bunnell Traveling Fellowship to Honduras and Cambodia. J Hand Surg 2004; 29(6):987–93.
12. Butler MW, Ozgediz D, Poenaru D, et al. The global paediatric surgery network: a model of subspecialty collaboration within global surgery. World J Surg 2015;39(2):335–42.
13. Martiniuk AL, Manouchehrian M, Negin JA, et al. Brain gains: a literature review of medical missions to low and middle-income countries. BMC Health Serv Res 2012;12(1).
14. Meier D. Opportunities and improvisations: a pediatric surgeon's suggestions for successful short-term surgical volunteer work in resource-poor areas. World J Surg 2010;34(5):941–6.
15. Schneider WJ, Migliori MR, Gosain AK, et al. Volunteers in plastic surgery guidelines for providing surgical care for children in the less developed world: part II. Ethical considerations. Plast Reconstr Surg 2011;128(3):216e–22e.
16. Wolfberg AJ. Volunteering overseas — lessons from surgical brigades. N Engl J Med 2006;354(5):443–5.
17. Kozin SH. The richness of caring for the poor: the development and implementation of the touching hands project. J Hand Surg 2015;40(3):566–75.
18. Grimes CE, Maraka J, Kingsnorth AN, et al. Guidelines for surgeons on establishing projects in low-income countries. World J Surg 2013;37(6):1203–7.
19. Canizares MF, Rios Roque JJ, Ramos Zelaya G, et al. Assessment of health needs in children with congenital upper limb differences in nicaragua: community case study. Front Public Health 2017;5:123.
20. Orser BA, Suresh S, Evers AS. SmartTots update regarding anesthetic neurotoxicity in the developing brain. Anesth Analg 2018;126(4):1393.
21. Gawande A. The checklist manifesto: how to get things right. New York: Henry Holt and Company; 2010.
22. Haynes AB, Weiser TG, Berry WR, et al. A surgical safety checklist to reduce morbidity and mortality in a global population. N Engl J Med 2009;360(5): 491–9.
23. Manske MCB, Rios Roque JJ, Zelaya GR, et al. Pediatric hand surgery training in nicaragua: a sustainable model of surgical education in a resource-poor environment. Front Public Health 2017;5:75.
24. Chung KY. Plastic and reconstructive surgery in global health: let's reconstruct global surgery. Plast Reconstr Surg Glob Open 2017;5(4):e1273.
25. James MA, Bagley AM, Brasington K, et al. Impact of prostheses on function and quality of life for children with unilateral congenital below-the-elbow deficiency. J Bone Joint Surg Am 2006;88(11):2356–65.
26. Goodell PB, Bauer AS, Oishi S, et al. Functional assessment of children and adolescents with symbrachydactyly: a unilateral hand malformation. J Bone Joint Surg 2017;99(13):1119.
27. Ezaki M, Oishi SN. Technique of forearm osteotomy for pediatric problems. J Hand Surg 2012;37(11): 2400–3.
28. Bamshad M, Van Heest AE, Pleasure D. Arthrogryposis: a review and update. J Bone Joint Surg Am 2009;91(Suppl 4):40–6.
29. Van Heest A, James MA, Lewica A, et al. Posterior Elbow capsulotomy with triceps lengthening for treatment of elbow extension contracture in children with arthrogryposis. J Bone Joint Surg Am 2008; 90(7):1517–23.
30. Foy CA, Mills J, Wheeler L, et al. Long-term outcome following carpal wedge osteotomy in the arthrogrypotic patient. J Bone Jt Surg 2013;95(20):e150.
31. Ezaki M, Oishi SN. Index rotation flap for palmar thumb release in arthrogryposis. Tech Hand Up Extrem Surg 2010;14(1):38–40.
32. Jackson TJ, Shah AS, Arkader A. Is routine spine MRI necessary in skeletally immature patients with MHE? identifying patients at risk for spinal osteochondromas. J Pediatr Orthop 2019;39(2):e147–52.

33. Klein C, Delcourt T, Salon A, et al. Surgical treatment of enchondromas of the hand during childhood in ollier disease. J Hand Surg 2018;43(10):946.e1-5.

34. Smith BW, Daunter AK, Yang LJ-S, et al. An update on the management of neonatal brachial plexus palsy—replacing old paradigms: a review. JAMA Pediatr 2018;172(6):585–91.

35. Hale HB, Bae DS, Waters PM. Current concepts in the management of brachial plexus birth palsy. J Hand Surg 2010;35(2):322–31.

36. Bauer AS, Lucas JF, Heyrani N, et al. Ultrasound screening for posterior shoulder dislocation in infants with persistent brachial plexus birth palsy. J Bone Jt Surg 2017;99(9):778–83.

37. Buchanan PJ, Grossman JAI, Price AE, et al. The use of botulinum toxin injection for brachial plexus birth injuries: a systematic review of the literature. HAND 2019;14(2):150–4.

38. Pearl M, Edgerton B, Kazimiroff P, et al. Arthroscopic release and latissimus dorsi transfer for shoulder internal rotation contractures and glenohumeral deformity secondary to brachial plexus birth palsy. J Bone Joint Surg Am 2006;88(3):564–74.

39. Anderson KA, O'Dell MA, James MA. Shoulder external rotation tendon transfers for brachial plexus birth palsy. Tech Hand Up Extrem Surg 2006;10(2):60.

40. Waters PM, Bae DS. The effect of derotational humeral osteotomy on global shoulder function in brachial plexus birth palsy. J Bone Joint Surg Am 2006;88(5):1035–42.

41. DeDeugd CM, Shin AY, Shaughnessy WJ. Derotational pronation-producing osteotomy of the radius and biceps tendon rerouting for supination contractures in neonatal brachial plexus palsy patients. Tech Hand Up Extrem Surg 2018;22(1):10–4.

42. Van Heest AE, Bagley A, Molitor F, et al. Tendon transfer surgery in upper-extremity cerebral palsy is more effective than botulinum toxin injections or regular, ongoing therapy. J Bone Joint Surg Am 2015;97(7):529–36.

43. James M, Bagley A, Vogler J, et al. Correlation between standard upper extremity impairment measures and activity-based function testing in upper extremity cerebral palsy. J Pediatr Orthop 2017; 37(2):102–6.

44. Donadio J, Upex P, Bachy M, et al. Wrist arthrodesis in adolescents with cerebral palsy. J Hand Surg Eur Vol 2016;41(7):758–62.

45. Gupta RK, Jindal N, Kamboj K. Neglected post burns contracture of hand in children: analysis of contributory socio-cultural factors and the impact of neglect on outcome. J Clin Orthop Trauma 2014;5(4):215–20.

Treating Hand Trauma in Low-Resource Setting
A Challenge for Low- and Middle-Income Countries

Kate Elzinga, MD[a],*, Kevin C. Chung, MD, MS[b]

KEYWORDS

- Global surgery • Hand surgery • Limited resources • Low- and middle-income countries
- Surgical education • Surgical simulation

KEY POINTS

- Hand trauma is common in low- and middle-income countries. Health policy changes have the greatest potential to reduce patient morbidity.
- Hand surgery education in low- and middle-income countries is best delivered using a combination of in-person teaching, written resources, videos, and Internet and social media platforms.
- Surgical simulation is a valuable tool for training worldwide. New technologies can be used at no cost in low- and middle-income countries to facilitate medical education while providing feedback to learners.

INTRODUCTION

The Lancet Commission on Global Surgery has determined that 90% of patients in low- and middle-income countries (LMICs) cannot access basic surgical care.[1] The lack of access to surgical care affects 5 billion people worldwide. More lives are lost annually because of conditions requiring surgical care (16.9 million) than from human immunodeficiency virus/AIDS (1.5 million), tuberculosis (1.2 million), and malaria (1.2 million) combined.[1] Although hand trauma is not typically life-threatening, hand injuries have a high rate of morbidity. Hand trauma often results in a decreased quality of life; compromise of a patient's ability to work and to contribute to their community; and in some cases, the inability to care for one's self, particularly in cases of severe bilateral hand injuries. Children often receive priority for treatment of hand injuries because of their increased risk of trauma and their potential for improved outcomes compared with adults.[2]

Hand trauma is common in LMICs. A patient's dominant hand is most often affected, worsening the prognosis for the patient's return to work. Common causes of hand trauma include traffic accidents (vehicular and pedestrian injuries), occupational accidents, burns, falls, weapons (guns, machetes, landmines, bombs), interpersonal conflicts and ethnoreligious clashes, and terrorism.[3] Motorcycles are commonly used for transportation and are often poorly maintained, road infrastructure is insufficient, traffic laws are poorly enforced, and protective gear is absent resulting in numerous accidents and hand injuries on a daily

Disclosure Statement: The authors have nothing to disclose.
[a] Section of Plastic Surgery, University of Calgary, South Health Campus, 4448 Front St SE, Calgary, Alberta T3M 1M4, Canada; [b] Section of Plastic Surgery, The University of Michigan Medical School, The University of Michigan Health System, 1500 East Medical Center Drive, 2130 Taubman Center, SPC 5340, Ann Arbor, MI 48109-0340, USA
* Corresponding author.
E-mail address: kate.elzinga@ahs.ca

Hand Clin 35 (2019) 479–486
https://doi.org/10.1016/j.hcl.2019.07.012

basis. Occupational accidents are frequent; protective clothing, machine safeguards, and return to work programs are commonly absent in LMICs.

Limited access to health care in LMICs results in untreated hand injuries that can lead to a marked decrease in function and chronic pain because they do not heal well by secondary intention. Hand therapy is rare; stiff joints and contractures are common. When surgery is performed, postoperative rehabilitation is rarely available and often inaccessible to patients, leading to suboptimal outcomes.

Providing education to LMICs on the treatment of hand injuries to create a safe, sustainable system for the care of hand trauma patients is paramount. Hand surgery is a multidisciplinary field. In addition to training surgeons to provide operative care, training anesthesiologists, nurses, and therapists in the care of these injuries is critical for optimizing outcomes. Anesthesia guidelines for children are particularly important for patient safely.[4] This article outlines some of the challenges faced by LMICs in caring for hand trauma patients.

HEALTH CARE POLICY

To decrease the morbidity of hand injuries in LMICs, prevention is of the greatest importance. Policy changes have a larger impact on population health compared with augmenting the number of medical professionals available. Surgeons and allied health care workers play an important part in patient advocacy and health care policy change.[5,6] Mandating the use of helmets and protective clothing and enforcing regular vehicle maintenance inspections prevents injuries and lessens their severity. Requiring workplace safety policies and increasing management engagement in safety results in improved mental and physical health of workers.[7]

GLOBAL HAND SURGERY EDUCATION

Teaching knowledge, skills, and decision-making permits providers in LMICs to care for patients who sustain hand trauma (**Fig. 1**). A flexible, multidimensional education delivery system is important to permit ongoing learning. In-person, video, and written forms of teaching each provide benefit to learners.[8] Resources, such as textbooks, journal articles, and instructional videos that permit self-directed learning, and timely review of materials when cases arise are valuable in LMICs. The goal is to educate and empower local surgeons, allied health care professionals, hospitals, and communities in the care of hand trauma patients.[9]

The increasing access to social media worldwide has had major benefits for global medical education, permitting sharing of educational resources and real-time discussion between health care providers.[10] It is particularly helpful for providers in training and professionals early in their careers to have access to experts to review cases and discuss treatment options immediately via online forums. Pictures and videos can be shared, with the appropriate patient permission, to facilitate communication. Multiple treatment options can be sought from health care providers across the world and then the most appropriate treatment implemented based on the available resources. Mentorship can be provided to health care professionals working in geographically isolated areas.

Archived videos, didactic teaching Web casts, and live surgical demonstrations permit thousands of surgeons to review the care of hand trauma injuries. Educational Web sites, such as Hand-e created by the American Society for Surgery of the Hand (https://www.assh.org/Hand-e), can provide free or low-cost access to thousands of peer-reviewed articles, presentations, and videos to those working in LMICs.

Some studies have shown that high-resource teaching methods (expert instruction) do not have a statistically significant benefit over low-resource methods (video and lectures).[11] The use of video can permit learners to review material as frequently as desired and can reach a large global audience. Videos can be created in LMICs by filming when experts are present, creating an archive of material useful to current and future learners.

Surgical Missions

An analysis of 22 surgical missions performed from 2015 to 2017 in eight different countries revealed that plastic surgery is economically sustainable in LMICs with interventions considered to be cost-effective or very-cost-effective as per the World Health Organization guidelines.[12–14]

Surgeons and their teams can travel to LMICs to effectively deliver care and education. Occasionally, acute trauma patients benefit from their care if the timing of their injury coincides with the arrival of the team. More commonly, surgical treatment of patients with congenital hand deformities and chronic hand injuries as a result of trauma are the focus of the visiting teams. Providing didactic lectures to the local care providers permits visiting educators to extrapolate from the patients cared for during their trip to future patients who will present with acute hand trauma. Presentations are given to local physicians with an emphasis on injuries seen in their region. Questions are

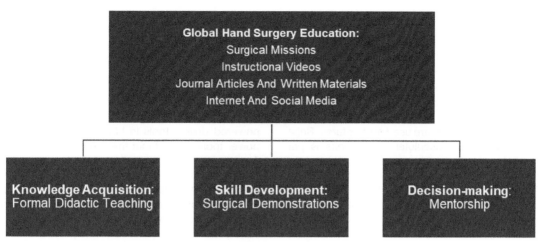

Fig. 1. Multifaceted approach to global hand surgery education.

encouraged to provide directed advice about patient problems that are frequently encountered. Case discussions can help learners apply the knowledge provided in the didactic lecture to patient cases.

Kozin[15] has stated that a bilateral exchange between the visiting surgical team and host country is necessary "emphasizing patient care, education, resource management, and research." Engaging local surgeons, residents, medical students, nurses, and therapists is often a key priority of visiting health care professionals to improve the delivery of future, sustainable hand trauma care in LMICs. The transmission of skills, knowledge, and techniques permits future generations of patients to benefit from the care provided by local physicians and allied health care professionals.

Creating a curriculum for teaching the principles of care in hand trauma provides learners with knowledge using an organized approach.[16] It permits multiple teachers to participate in the teaching while ensuring that all topics are covered. Providing learners with precourse materials including journal articles, textbook chapters, videos, and World Wide Web–based materials permits learners to prepare. They can review the basics of hand anatomy, trauma injury patterns, and treatment goals in advance so that their time with visiting teachers is used for case discussions and question-and-answer sessions.

Academic partnerships between universities in LMICs and high-income countries can permit formalized, ongoing training support in countries where this training would otherwise be unavailable. Providing education to surgeons in their country of origin can limit the "brain drain" created by capable physicians leaving to practice in other countries. Permitting local physicians to pursue postgraduate degrees in their home country facilitates their ability to care for patients in their country.

Train the Trainer

In "train the trainer" programs, students are taught the essentials of hand trauma care and then can teach others.[17,18] These models are more sustainable than relying on visiting teachers on an ongoing basis. Teaching emphasis is placed on hand surgery procedures that are inexpensive, reliable, and effective.[19]

Permitting LMICs to become independent in providing surgical care is the ultimate goal. Surgical volunteer organizations can provide care for patients with chronic stable hand deformities, but acute trauma care can only be delivered in a timely fashion by local surgeons. Building local competency and capacity must be achieved.[20] Providing algorithms can facilitate decision-making and triaging. Support must be available for local providers when outcomes deviate from the expected. With increasing access to free social media and Internet-based text-messaging and video services, surgeons in LMICs have improved timely access to surgeons in other parts of the world who can provide timely advice and guidance on patient care.

Principles of Hand Trauma

Emphasis is placed on teaching the principles of hand trauma. These principles permit providers to apply their knowledge to subsequent simple and complex patient problems in an organized fashion. Initial Advanced Trauma Life Support protocols are reviewed, emphasizing life over limb. After the primary survey, the limbs are assessed in the secondary survey and initial treatment including reduction, splinting, and decontamination is started for hand injuries. Radiograph is the mainstay of imaging for hand trauma, in low-, middle-, and high-income countries.

Thorough debridement is essential to the patient's overall outcome. Devitalized tissue is removed to prevent infection. Stable fixation and early range of motion are used for fractures. Rehabilitation of the musculotendinous units is performed under the guidance of a therapist or the surgeon. Soft tissue coverage is typically performed with skin grafts or pedicled flaps. Range of motion precautions and protective splinting are important following the repair of tendon and arterial injuries.

Simulation

Simulation has been applied to several different fields including military, aviation, automobile, city planning, sport, and biomechanical industries.[21] It has been successfully used in all areas of medicine including surgery, anesthesiology, emergency medicine, obstetrics, and pediatrics. Simulation is useful for teaching procedural skills, including those required for hand surgery. Low cost, portability, and validity are important.[22] Simulation programs in such countries as Rwanda have demonstrated its benefits in surgical training with the most benefit derived by junior-level learners.[23]

Technology simulation

As smart phones become more widespread, technological simulations available through free applications, such as Touch Surgery (www.touchsurgery.com), can provide learners with an opportunity to rehearse a particular surgery in advance until they are comfortable performing the procedure under guidance of their preceptor.[24] Simulation can provide an excellent review for experienced surgeons who may perform certain procedures infrequently. Touch Surgery permits surgeons to practice more than 160 procedures, including hand surgery procedures with acute and elective case demonstrations, such as carpal tunnel release, local flap and skin graft closure, carpometacarpal joint arthroplasty of the thumb, thumb ulnar collateral ligament repair, scaphoid and distal radius open reduction and internal fixation, syndactyly release, trigger finger and de Quervain release, tendon repair, lag screw and tension band fixation, and Dupuytren. Anatomy and surgical approaches are also included. The app details the steps of the procedure, the equipment required, and permits self-testing.

Simulation tools are particularly useful for less-experienced surgeons. As digital content continues to emerge, LMICs will have greater access to free content with high educational impact.[25] Simulation must be guided by the resources available at the local hospital. For example, performing simulation with plate and screw techniques is often of little value if only K-wires are available for fracture fixation. Furthermore, K-wires are often placed with hand-powered drilling tools in LMICs rather than with power tools and without the use of intraoperative fluoroscopy. Hammering is a useful technique for K-wire insertion in LMICs and has been shown to be superior to drilling with faster insertion times and less thermal damage.[26] Drill covers are an innovative solution to permit inexpensive hardware store drills to be used sterilely for hardware placement (https://arbutusmedical.ca/human-health/products/products/). If simulation content is produced based on the resources and equipment available in LMICs, the simulation is of highest utility to the local surgeons.

Bone simulation

Synthetic bone models, created from plastics and epoxies, such as Sawbones (Pacific Research Laboratories, Vashon, WA), Synbone (Malans, Switzerland), and Promedicus (Mikołów ul. Brzoskwiniowa, Poland), are a useful tool for simulation.[27] The increased number of vendors producing these products has reduced costs and improved access.[28] Artificial soft tissue coverage is added to increase the complexity of the simulation. This can permit learners the opportunity to review anatomy and to practice surgical landmarking. This is particularity valuable for surgeons working without intraoperative fluoroscopy where tactile feedback is critical for placing K-wires. Joint aspiration simulation is effectively practiced using Sawbones.[29]

Microsurgery simulation

Nonliving models reduce cost and resources needed for microsurgical training. Microscopes are frequently unavailable in LMICs. iPad trainers have been shown to permit early microsurgical skill acquisition comparable with practice under a microscope.[30] A low-cost jeweler's microscope has shown equivalent outcomes compared with surgical microscopes.

Loupe magnification, microsurgery instruments, and nonsterile gauze is effectively used for practice.[27] The learner passes a suture above and below adjacent threads of the gauze. The gauze can be purchased in bulk to reduce costs. Latex gloves are used for practicing knot placement and tying. Once the learner feels comfortable with the instruments and passing and tying the sutures, a vessel can be anastomosed. Chicken vessels are practical models.[31] The brachial artery located in a chicken wing approximates the size of a digital artery. Chicken legs permit practice on the femoral artery, vein, and sciatic nerve. Learners can improve their microsurgical skills in a controlled setting, improving their ability to care for subsequent injured patients, such as those requiring digital nerve or artery repair following a hand injury.

HAND TRAUMA TREATMENT PRINCIPLES

Hand traumas are often complex and require multidisciplinary treatment to optimize aesthetic and functional outcomes. Wound care is an integral component of treatment to prevent infection, joint contracture, and scarring. Early range of motion, ideally supervised by a therapist, permits patients to return to their activities of daily living and work quicker. Preventing long-term injury morbidity is facilitated by patient education, which permits patients to play an active role in their care. For patients with severe injuries (eg, those resulting in amputations), learning functional adaptations can permit patients to perform their daily tasks in new ways to maintain their independence

and their ability to contribute to the well-being of their families and communities. Wound care, hand therapy, patient education, and early return to recreational and occupational activities improve patients' short- and long-term outcomes (**Fig. 2**).

WOUND CARE

In LMICs, access to purified water is often lacking. If access to safe drinking water is available, this water is used to cleanse wounds from hand trauma directly. Basic soap and clean dressings are used. Sterile dressings are not necessary; their additional cost is often prohibitive in LMICs and basic dressing materials have comparable sterility.[32]

Permitting wounds to heal by secondary intention results in the ingrowth of sensate and durable skin coverage with minimal hypersensitivity and cold intolerance.[33] To facilitate wound healing, wounds should be kept clean and moist. A simple petroleum ointment suffices. Coverage with a reusable, flexible dressing, such as Coban, permits the maintenance of a clean, moist wound-healing environment while permitting joint range of motion and compression to minimize edema. Coban and similar outer coverage dressings are

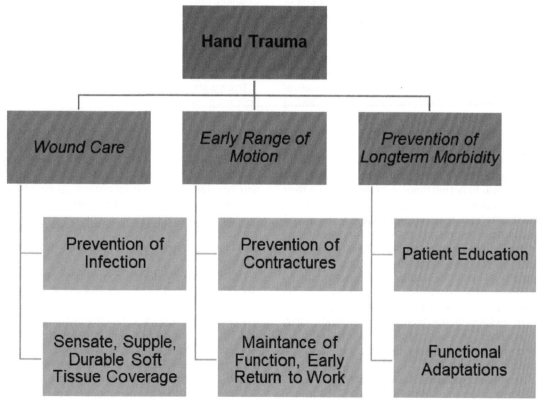

Fig. 2. Treatment principles for hand trauma.

applied directly to the wound over the petroleum ointment, minimizing the complexity of the dressing. Gauze is not required. Patients can learn how to apply the dressing quickly and easily themselves.

Permitting secondary intention wound healing is used for wounds with exposed bone, exposed tendon, and over joints with excellent results. Contracture of an open wound over an amputation stump permits durable healing. Hygiene is of critical importance during the secondary intention healing process. If infection occurs, wound healing stalls and debridement may be needed. Permitting injured workers to return to work early with protective dressings can minimize their financial hardship from missed work while protecting open wounds from the environment.

If joints become stiff or contracted from secondary healing without adequate joint mobilization, resurfacing of defects with nonmicrovascular flaps is performed. Pedicled flaps from the chest, abdomen, or groin can restore supple soft tissue coverage following hand injuries.[34]

EARLY RANGE OF MOTION

Joint contractures are a major issue in LMICs. Splinting material and expertise are often deficient. After injury, which is often resulting from trauma or burns, the metacarpophalangeal joints are held in extension because this position accommodates greater edema. In turn, the flexor tension on the interphalangeal joints increases, whereas the extensor tension decreases, leading to flexion of the interphalangeal joints. This intrinsic negative/minus position of the hand results in shortening of the collateral ligaments and volar plates of the interphalangeal joints, joint contractures, and loss of range of motion.

Patients should guide their return to activities by their pain. They should quickly wean off of all pain medication to permit them to safely increase their activities over time while listening to their body for feedback from their injury. Patients should be encouraged to do early active and passive range of motion exercises to mobilize fluids out of their joints, to preserve mobility, and to prevent disuse atrophy. Range of motion exercises can be demonstrated to patients and their families by physicians, nurses, and other allied health professions quickly at the time of the patient's initial assessment. If hand fractures are present, as long as they are stable, early active range of motion is performed.

Unstable fractures require internal (often K-wires) or external (often splinting) stabilization. Typically, the joint above and below the fracture must be immobilized until the fracture becomes stable by early callous formation. Repeat radiograph imaging may not be available, so decreasing tenderness at the fracture site is used to guide weaning from splints and increasing range of motion. Range of motion of unaffected joints is commenced immediately.

Minimizing the length of time K-wires are used reduces the risk of soft tissue and bone infection. K-wires can often be removed from finger fractures after 2.5 weeks and from distal radius fractures after 4 weeks.[35] The patient can then advance their rehabilitative range of motion exercises. Prophylactic antibiotics are not typically indicated and the K-wires are left outside the skin to facilitate their removal in clinic without anesthesia, which decreases costs for the patient.

PREVENTION OF LONG-TERM MORBIDITY

As noted hand surgeon Pulvertaft[36] wrote, surgery of the hand can only be successful if "the surgery is precise and the aftercare is unrelenting." Educating and engaging patients in their care from the onset of their injury improves their self-efficacy and overall outcome.[37] Teaching family members how to assist patients with wound cleaning, dressing placement, and range of motion exercises, particularly for patients requiring assistance, such as children and the elderly, decreases the demand on limited health care personnel and reduces health care system and direct patient costs.

Transportation is a major issue in LMICs. Follow-up appointments can cause an undue burden on patients if they need to miss work, walk long distances or find transportation, and/or arrange childcare. Every effort is made to communicate the required wound care, therapy exercises, plan for return of activity and work, and long-term prognosis for patients at their initial visit in case follow-up appointments are not feasible. Patients or their accompanying family members and friends should be encouraged to take notes during the consultation for future reference.

Often within a patient's community, other people who have had similar injuries exist. Although advice must be interpreted with some caution, guidance and encouragement are beneficial to patients in the acute phase of their injury, particularly when others in the community have recovered well and have little-to-no pain or functional impairments. Connecting with multiple patients can provide patients with a greater spectrum of reference and aid in their postinjury recovery.

Upper Extremity Amputations

Prostheses are rarely available in LMICs. They are expensive, lack durability, require regular maintenance and replacement, and need to be refitted frequently. They are often damaged in labor jobs. Maintenance of upper extremity length and as many joints as possible is critical for maintaining a patient's ability to perform self-care and for employment. A transradial, below-elbow amputation is far more functional than a transhumeral, above-elbow amputation. The additional length of the arm and preservation of the elbow joint improves the patient's ability to carry and manipulate objects. Permitting wounds to heal by secondary intention to preserve length is favored rather than early shortening, debridement, and closure following an upper extremity amputation.

SUMMARY

Overall, the goal of health care is to prevent injury, minimize disability, and promote wellness, at home and abroad.[38] Effective, consistent longitudinal services are required and must be easily accessible to patients. Developing curriculum to help train local physicians can aid LMICs in providing care for patients with hand injuries.

Short-term surgical trips to LMICs can benefit a limited number of patients through the surgical care provided by the visiting team and can reach a far greater number of patients through the teaching provided to the local health care providers. Didactic lectures, surgical demonstrations, and access to expert surgeons via the Internet for mentorship and help with decision-making can permit knowledge and skill acquisition by local surgeons to benefit patients for years to come.[39]

REFERENCES

1. Meara JG, Leather AJ, Hagander L, et al. Global surgery 2030: evidence and solutions for achieving health, welfare, and economic development. Int J Obstet Anesth 2016;25:75–8.
2. Chung KY, Hanemaayer A, Poenaru D. Pediatric hand surgery in global health: the role for international outreach. Ann Plast Surg 2017;78(2):162–70.
3. Adoga AA, Ozoilo KN. The epidemiology and type of injuries seen at the accident and emergency unit of a Nigerian referral center. J Emerg Trauma Shock 2014;7(2):77–82.
4. Schneider WJ, Migliori MR, Gosain AK, et al. Volunteers in plastic surgery guidelines for providing surgical care for children in the less developed world: part II. Ethical considerations. Plast Reconstr Surg 2011;128(3):216e–22e.
5. Sethi MK, Obremskey A, Sathiyakumar V, et al. The evolution of advocacy and orthopaedic surgery. Clin Orthop Relat Res 2013;471(6):1873–8.
6. Dadzie G, Aziato L, Aikins AD. "We are the best to stand in for patients": a qualitative study on nurses' advocacy characteristics in Ghana. BMC Nurs 2017;16:61.
7. Kiani F, Khodabakhsh MR. Preventing injuries in workers: the role of management practices in decreasing injuries reporting. Int J Health Policy Manag 2014;3(4):171–7.
8. Kemp N, Grieve R. Face-to-face or face-to-screen? Undergraduates' opinions and test performance in classroom vs. online learning. Front Psychol 2014; 5:1278.
9. Chung KY. The role for international outreach in hand surgery. J Hand Surg Am 2017;42(8):652–5.
10. Kwon SH, Goh R, Wang ZT, et al. Tips for making a successful online microsurgery educational platform: the experience of international microsurgery club. Plast Reconstr Surg 2019;143(1):221e–33e.
11. Bhashyam AR, Logan C, Roberts HJ, et al. A randomized controlled pilot study of educational techniques in teaching basic arthroscopic skills in a low-income country. Arch Bone Jt Surg 2017; 5(2):82–8.
12. Nasser JS, Billig JI, Sue GR, et al. Evaluating the economic sustainability of plastic and reconstructive surgical efforts in the developing world. Plast Reconstr Surg Glob Open 2018;6(8S):194–5.
13. Baltussen RM, Adam T, Tan-Torres Edejer T, et al. Making choices in health: WHO guide to cost-effectiveness analysis 2003. Available at: https://www.who.int/choice/publications/p_2003_generalised_cea.pdf.
14. Qiu X, Nasser JS, Sue GR, et al. Cost-effectiveness analysis of humanitarian hand surgery trips according to WHO-CHOICE thresholds. J Hand Surg Am 2019;44(2):93–103.
15. Kozin SH. Commentary on "the role for international outreach in hand surgery". J Hand Surg Am 2017; 42(8):656.
16. Chung KY. Plastic and reconstructive surgery in global health: let's reconstruct global surgery. Plast Reconstr Surg Glob Open 2017;5(4):e1273.
17. Lucchini RG, McDiarmid M, Van der Laan G, et al. Education and training: key factors in global occupational and environmental health. Ann Glob Health 2018;84(3):436–41.
18. König S, Stieger P, Sippel S, et al. Train-the-trainer: professionalisation of didactics in daily clinical routine. The personal perception of clinical teaching staff with respect to didactic competence and the framework conditions of teaching. Zentralbl Chir 2019 [Epub ahead of print]. [in German].

19. Marseille E, Morshed S. Essential surgery is cost effective in resource-poor countries. Lancet Glob Health 2014;2(6):e302–3.

20. Aliu O, Corlew SD, Heisler ME, et al. Building surgical capacity in low-resource countries: a qualitative analysis of task shifting from surgeon volunteers' perspectives. Ann Plast Surg 2014;72(1):108–12.

21. Singh H, Kalani M, Acosta-Torres S, et al. History of simulation in medicine: from Resusci Annie to the Ann Myers Medical Center. Neurosurgery 2013; 73(Suppl 1):9–14.

22. Wiet GJ, Stredney D, Kerwin T, et al. Simulation for training in resource-restricted countries: using a scalable temporal bone surgical simulator. Int J Med Educ 2016;7:293–4.

23. Tansley G, Bailey JG, Gu Y, et al. Efficacy of surgical simulation training in a low-income country. World J Surg 2016;40(11):2643–9.

24. Tulipan J, Miller A, Park AG, et al. Touch surgery: analysis and assessment of validity of a hand surgery simulation "app". Hand (N Y) 2019;14(3):311–6.

25. Nicolosi F, Rossini Z, Zaed I, et al. Neurosurgical digital teaching in low-middle income countries: beyond the frontiers of traditional education. Neurosurg Focus 2018;45(4):E17.

26. Franssen BB, Schuurman AH, Brouha PC, et al. Hammering K-wires is superior to drilling with irrigation. Hand (N Y) 2009;4(2):108–12.

27. Reed JD, Stanbury SJ, Menorca RM, et al. The emerging utility of composite bone models in biomechanical studies of the hand and upper extremity. J Hand Surg Am 2013;38(3):583–7.

28. Hetaimish BM. Sawbones laboratory in orthopedic surgical training. Saudi Med J 2016;37(4):348–53.

29. Sterrett AG, Bateman H, Guthrie J, et al. Virtual rheumatology: using simulators and a formal workshop to teach medical students, internal medicine residents, and rheumatology subspecialty residents arthrocentesis. J Clin Rheumatol 2011;17(3):121–3.

30. Malik MM, Hachach-Haram N, Tahir M, et al. Acquisition of basic microsurgery skills using home-based simulation training: a randomised control study. J Plast Reconstr Aesthet Surg 2017;70(4):478–86.

31. Singh M, Ziolkowski N, Ramachandran S, et al. Development of a five-day basic microsurgery simulation training course: a cost analysis. Arch Plast Surg 2014;41(3):213–7.

32. Alqahtani M, Lalonde DH. Sterile versus nonsterile clean dressings. Can J Plast Surg 2006;14(1):25–7.

33. Krauss EM, Lalonde DH. Secondary healing of fingertip amputations: a review. Hand (N Y) 2014; 9(3):282–8.

34. Naalla R, Chauhan S, Dave A, et al. Reconstruction of post-traumatic upper extremity soft tissue defects with pedicled flaps: an algorithmic approach to clinical decision making. Chin J Traumatol 2018;21(6):338–51.

35. Subramanian P, Kantharuban S, Shilston S, et al. Complications of Kirschner-wire fixation in distal radius fractures. Tech Hand Up Extrem Surg 2012; 16(3):120–3.

36. Pulvertaft G. Hand surgery in developing countries. Ann Chir Main 1987;6(4):329–31.

37. Paterick TE, Patel N, Tajik AJ, et al. Improving health outcomes through patient education and partnerships with patients. Proc (Bayl Univ Med Cent) 2017;30(1):112–3.

38. Yuan F, Chung KC. Defining quality in health care and measuring quality in surgery. Plast Reconstr Surg 2016;137(5):1635–44.

39. Chung KC, Billig JI, Nasser JS. Educating hand surgeons in the developing world: where do we go from here? J Hand Surg Eur Vol 2019;44(2):221–2.

A Systematic Review of Orthopedic Global Outreach Efforts Based on WHO-CHOICE Thresholds

Michael T. Nolte, MD[a], Jacob S. Nasser, BS[b], Kevin C. Chung, MD, MS[c],*

KEYWORDS

- Cost-effectiveness analysis • WHO-CHOICE • Global surgery • Orthopedic hand surgery
- Economic analysis

KEY POINTS

- The most common intervention in the cost-effectiveness analyses included in this study was fracture fixation, followed by wound debridement, amputation, and contracture release.
- All the orthopedic interventions were found to be *very cost-effective* according to WHO-CHOICE thresholds.
- Orthopedic outreach has potential to be universally very cost-effective. Efforts to establish infrastructure through training are particularly valuable.
- The findings of this review should encourage directed funding and devoted resources toward future orthopedic global health efforts.

INTRODUCTION

Injuries and musculoskeletal disorders accounted for just less than 5 million deaths and 16% of the world's burden of disease according to the World Health Organization (WHO) in 2015.[1] Injury in particular is a major health concern that disproportionately affects low- and middle-income countries (LMIC), with an estimated 80% to 90% of all injury-related deaths occurring in LMICs. Furthermore, for every death caused by injury, there is an estimated 20 to 50 nonfatal injuries that result in disability and decreased quality of life.[2] Similarly, musculoskeletal disorders unrelated to injury pose a substantial risk to productivity and financial security. An estimated $8 trillion of cumulative gross domestic product will be lost worldwide over the next 15 years from decreased economic productivity attributable to musculoskeletal disorder and injury, with losses 50% greater in LMICs than high-income countries.[3]

In response to the growing need for surgery in the developing world, there has been an increased interest in subspecialty surgical outreach. An

Funding: This work was supported by a Midcareer Investigator Award in Patient-Oriented Research (2 K24-AR053120-06) to K.C. Chung. The content is solely the responsibility of the authors and does not necessarily represent the official views of the National Institutes of Health.

Disclosure Statement: The authors did not have any relationship with a commercial company with a financial interest in the subject discussed in this article.

[a] Department of Orthopaedic Surgery, Rush University Medical Center, 1653 West Congress Parkway, Chicago, IL 60612, USA; [b] Department of Surgery, Section of Plastic Surgery, University of Michigan Medical School, 2800 Plymouth Road, Building 14 G200, Ann Arbor, MI 48109, USA; [c] Section of Plastic Surgery, University of Michigan Medical School, The University of Michigan Health System, 1500 East Medical Center Drive, 2130 Taubman Center, SPC 5340, Ann Arbor, MI 48109-5340, USA

* Corresponding author.

E-mail address: kecchung@med.umich.edu

increasing number of surgical teams have completed trips to LMICs with the goal of providing a high volume of surgery to a local population over a short period of time or helping to educate local surgeons and establish infrastructure. The clinical scope of these outreach efforts is broad, ranging from fracture reduction and fixation to peripheral nerve repair.[4] The total expenditures for these trips can be substantial, ranging anywhere from $10 thousand to well greater than $1 million, depending on the location and extent of services provided.[4] Despite the best efforts of visiting surgeons, considerable need for surgical interventions remains after their departure. Orthopedic surgeons must therefore strive to use their expertise, time, and limited resources in outreach efforts both efficiently and cost-effectively.

The funding of outreach represents a sizable challenge with tremendous repercussions for patients and providers alike. Consider that from 1990 to 2014 approximately 458 billion dollars from public and private organizations were spent on global health efforts despite minimal availability of cost-effectiveness guidelines for interventions being performed.[5] In response to this challenge, WHO Choosing Interventions that are Cost-Effective initiative (WHO-CHOICE)[6] established detailed criteria for reporting, funding, and participating in medical and surgical outreach efforts around the world. A centerpiece of this initiative was the establishment of thresholds for determining the cost-effectiveness of specific efforts in LMICs. These thresholds specifically apply to the cost per Disability Adjusted Life Year (DALY) averted. The DALY is a statistical measure representing the number of years of life lost due to morbidity and mortality of a particular medical condition. The cost per DALY averted, therefore, is the amount of money that an intervention costs in order to successfully avert 1 year of life that would otherwise be lost to that morbidity and mortality. WHO-CHOICE applied the per capita gross domestic product (GDP) of the country in question as the threshold for "very cost-effective" and 3 times this level for "cost-effective." Similarly, an intervention with a cost per DALY averted of greater than 3 times the per capita GDP is considered to be "not cost-effective." In Ghana, for example, where the 2016 per-capita GDP is estimated to be $1513 dollars, an intervention that costs less than $1513 per DALY averted, such as caesarean section ($279 per DALY averted),[7] would be very cost-effective by WHO-CHOICE standards. Similarly, an intervention that costs between $1513 and $4539 per DALY averted in Ghana, such as glaucoma surgery ($1654 per DALY averted),[8] would be cost-effective but not

very cost-effective. Lastly, an intervention that costs greater than $2283 per DALY averted, or 3 times the per-capita GDP, such as breast cancer surveillance via routine mammography ($12,908 per DALY averted),[9] would be considered not cost-effective. Despite the exciting potential of these new guidelines, the value of published orthopedic interventions has yet to be uniformly analyzed in accordance with WHO-CHOICE thresholds.

In an effort to investigate the cost-effectiveness of orthopedic surgical outreach efforts, the authors systematically reviewed the literature on orthopedic surgical trips. They also analyzed the cost-effectiveness of efforts to train and educate orthopedic surgeons in LMICs, a growing area of outreach interest.[10,11] They aimed to determine the degree of cost-effectiveness according to WHO-CHOICE thresholds and to examine the specific type of orthopedic interventions being offered. The authors hypothesized that most of the published efforts in LMICs are considered very cost-effective by WHO-CHOICE standards, with an emphasis placed on trauma-related surgeries such as open reduction and internal fixations. They also hypothesized that outreach efforts that provided more trauma-related or emergent surgeries were generally more cost-effective than those providing care that was nonemergent or unrelated to trauma. Findings from this review sheds light on the cost-effectiveness of orthopedic outreach relative to other surgical subspecialties and can be used by orthopedic surgeons, policy makers, and third-party funders to guide future outreach efforts to LMICs. Furthermore, because most of the orthopedic surgeons share a basic common surgical skillset, these results may help guide the types of procedures performed such that the most cost-effective care is delivered.

MATERIALS AND METHODS
Literature Search

A systematic review of the literature was performed to identify all studies that featured an economic analysis of one or more surgical trip that specifically provided orthopedic-related care. Examples of this include fracture fixation following trauma, amputation, extremity wound debridement, and treatment of burned extremities. The authors followed the Preferred Reporting Items for Systematic reviews and Meta-Analyses (PRISMA) guidelines (**Table 1**).[12] They searched 3 databases (PubMed, EMBASE, and MEDLINE) for articles in English that featured an economic analysis of one or more orthopedic-related surgical trip. The initial search was for all publications

Table 1
PRISMA guidelines fulfilled in this review

Topic	Fulfilled?
Identified as a systematic review	Yes
Summary of background and methods	Yes
Rationale is identified	Yes
Objective is identified	Yes
Review protocol provided	Yes
Eligibility criteria given	Yes
Information sources reported	Yes
Search strategy reported	Yes
Study selection process reported	Yes
Data collection process reported	Yes
Data variables of interest reported and defined	Yes
Methods for assessing risk reported	Yes
Principal summary measures reported	Yes
Methods reported for synthesis of results	Yes
Methods for risk of bias	No
Methods for additional analyses explained	—
Study selection described	Yes
Characteristics of studies provided	Yes
Risk of bias within each study reported	No
Results of each study reported	Yes
Synthesized results reported	Yes
Risk assessments reported	No
Additional analysis reported	—
Main findings summarized	Yes
Limitations discussed	No
Interpretation of results	Yes
Sources of funding	Yes

Adapted from Moher D, Liberati A, Tetzlaff J, Altman DG. Preferred reporting items for systematic reviews and meta-analyses: the PRISMA statement. *Ann Intern Med.* Aug 18 2009;151(4):264-269, w264; with permission.

containing the words "trip" and "economic" and appropriate synonyms for each. These terms were expanded to include the corresponding Medical Subject Headings (MeSH) and EMTREE subject headings. The search was limited to peer-reviewed articles published in English after 1990. A complete search algorithm can be found in **Table 2**. After eliminating duplicates, 2 reviewers separately screened publications by reviewing complete abstracts to discard articles that were not relevant to the topic. The full text of each article meeting inclusion criteria was read. In addition, the references of each qualifying article produced by the search were manually screened to detect additional studies that met inclusion criteria.

Study Criteria

An article had to provide an economic analysis of an orthopedic surgery outreach effort in order to be included in the review process. Interventions were deemed to be orthopedic if they could be applied to ICD-10 diagnostic codes M00-M99, which describe diseases of the musculoskeletal system and connective tissue.[13] The authors specifically sought surgical, rather than nonsurgical, interventions. However, several nonsurgical interventions have been referenced in interest of comparison. Articles that contained both orthopedic and nonorthopedic interventions were included in the review, with only data from the orthopedic-specific interventions analyzed. If the cost-effectiveness of the orthopedic intervention was not analyzed separately from the nonorthopedic intervention, the study was included nonetheless for comparison, with appropriate clarification in the results.

Data Extraction and Analysis

For each article that met study criteria, data regarding author, journal, year of publication, geographic location, type of cost-effectiveness measure, cost per outcome, unit of outcome, and currency used were collected. For ease of analysis and comparison, all cost data were adjusted to 2016 USD values. Where available in the literature, data regarding specific orthopedic procedure categories were collected, both in raw number and the proportion of total procedures for that particular outreach effort. These subcategories included, but were not limited to, fracture fixation, amputation, wound debridement, burn surgery, soft tissue repair, and correction of congenital deformities.

Quality Assessment

The authors performed a quality assessment of the eligible articles using the Drummond questionnaire (**Table 3**), a 10-point checklist for economic evaluation of health care programs, while assessing the quality of each reviewed paper.[14] A *Yes*, *No*, or *Partially* was assigned to each item. *Yes* was given a score of 1, and *No* or *Partially* was given a score of 0. The items were tallied to give a composite score for each article.[15]

Table 2
Search algorithm for PubMed, EMBASE, and MEDLINE

Database	Algorithm
PubMed	("humanitarian medicine"[tiab] or "humanitarian medical"[tiab] or "humanitarian outreach"[tiab] or "humanitarian mission"[tiab] or "humanitarian missions"[tiab] or "humanitarian assistance"[tiab] or "volunteer outreach"[tiab] or "volunteer mission"[tiab] or "volunteer missions"[tiab] or "volunteer surgical"[tiab] or "medical volunteer"[tiab] or "medical volunteering"[tiab] or "charity outreach"[tiab] or "charity mission"[tiab] or "charity missions"[tiab] or "international mission"[tiab] or "international missions"[tiab] or "international outreach"[tiab] or "international medical"[tiab] or "international surgical"[tiab] or "international volunteer"[tiab] or "international cooperation"[tiab] or "medical outreach"[tiab] or "medical brigade"[tiab] or "medical brigades"[tiab] or "medical mission"[tiab] or "medical missions"[tiab] or "medical tourism"[tiab] or "medical service trip"[tiab] or "medical service trips"[tiab] or "medical trip"[tiab] or "medical trips"[tiab] or "medical humanitarian"[tiab] or "outreach mission"[tiab] or "outreach missions"[tiab] or "surgical mission"[tiab] or "surgical missions"[tiab] or "humanitarian surgical"[tiab] or "misson"[tiab] or "missions"[tiab] or "overseas volunteer surgical"[tiab] or "overseas volunteer medical"[tiab] or "Medical tourism"[mh] OR "Medical Missions, official"[mh]) AND ("economic"[tiab] OR "economics"[tiab] OR "economic analysis"[tiab] OR "economic study"[tiab] OR "economic evaluation"[tiab] OR "economic assessment"[tiab] OR ("cost"[tiab] AND "benefit"[tiab]) OR ("cost"[tiab] AND "effective"[tiab]) OR ("cost"[tiab] AND "effectiveness"[tiab]) or "Cost-Benefit Analysis"[mh]) AND ("english"[la] and "1990/01/01"[dp] : "3000" [dp]).
EMBASE	((humanitarian OR volunteer or charity) NEAR/6 (medicine OR medical OR outreach OR mission*) or (international) NEAR/6 (mission* or outreach or volunteer*) OR (medical or surgical) NEAR/6 (volunteer* or outreach OR brigade* OR mission* OR tourism OR trip*) or 'Medical tourism'/exp) and ((economic* or cost*) NEAR/3 (benefit* or effective* or analysis or evaluation* or assessment*) or 'economic evaluation'/exp) AND ('english':la and [1990-2015]/py).
MEDLINE	(((((humanitarian OR volunteer* OR charity) adj6 (medicine OR medical OR outreach OR mission*)) OR ((international) adj6 (mission* or outreach or volunteer*)) OR ((medical OR surgical) adj6 (volunteer* OR outreach OR brigade* OR mission* OR tourism OR trip*))).mp) or (exp medical tourism/or exp medical missions, official/)) and ((((economic* or cost*) adj3 (benefit* or effective* or analysis or stud* or evaluation* or assessment*)).mp) or (exp cost-benefit analysis/)) and (english.la.)

RESULTS

Literature Review Findings

Of the 999 nonduplicate publications retrieved, 836 were eliminated after reading the title and abstract. Then the full text of the remaining 91 articles was comprehensively reviewed. Finally, 10 articles met the study criteria (**Fig. 1**). A brief summary of each article is provided in **Table 4**. Drummond questionnaire quality assessment suggested that all 10 articles had a score of 5 or greater, with a mean Drummond score of 6.4 (see **Table 3**).

Orthopedic Outreach Efforts

Each of the 10 eligible studies presented outreach efforts that featured orthopedic interventions (**Table 5**). Of these, 5 contained exclusively orthopedic interventions,[11,15–18] whereas 5 also analyzed obstetric[19] and general surgery[10,20–22] interventions. Africa was the most frequented

geographic region with 6 studies,[10,17,19–22] followed by Central America and the Caribbean.[15,16,18,21] The analysis period for these outreach efforts ranged in duration from 1 week to 2 years. Seven studies[10,17–22] represented efforts to contribute to infrastructure through training or through volunteering at an established hospital system, whereas 3 studies[11,15,16] describe short trips from visiting surgeons without explicit efforts to train local providers. Most of the studies analyzed efforts performed on an elective basis, with 2 studies[15,19] providing a comparison between emergent and elective outreach efforts.

Orthopedic Surgery Subspecialty Representation

Studies that provided a breakdown of orthopedic procedures by type are presented in **Table 6**, with the 3 most common procedures performed

Table 3
Drummond checklist for included studies

Author, Year	1	2	3	4	5	6	7	8	9	10	Total
Carlson et al,[18] 2012	•	•	•	•	•	•	•	•	•	•	7
Chen et al,[16] 2012	•	•	•	•	•	•	•	•	•	•	6
Gosselin et al,[20] 2006	•	•	•	•	•	•	•	•	•	•	6
Gosselin & Heitto,[10] 2008	•	•	•	•	•	•	•	•	•	•	7
Gosselin et al,[21] 2010	•	•	•	•	•	•	•	•	•	•	7
Gosselin et al,[15] 2011	•	•	•	•	•	•	•	•	•	•	6
Grimes et al,[17,34] 2014	•	•	•	•	•	•	•	•	•	•	5
Rattray et al,[22] 2013	•	•	•	•	•	•	•	•	•	•	7
Roberts et al,[19] 2016	•	•	•	•	•	•	•	•	•	•	8
Tadisina et al,[11] 2014	•	•	•	•	•	•	•	•	•	•	5

○, Yes; ●, No; ○, Unclear.

Drummond checklist questions: (1) Was a well-defined question posed in answerable form? (2) Was a comprehensive description of the competing alternatives given? (3) Was the effectiveness of the programs or services established? (4) Were all the important and relevant costs and consequences for each alternative identified? (5) Were costs and consequences measured accurately in appropriate physical units? (6) Were costs and consequences valued credibly? (7) Were costs and consequences adjusted for differential timing? (8) Was an incremental analysis of costs and consequences of alternatives performed? (9) Was allowance made for uncertainty in the estimates of costs and consequences? (10) Did the presentation and discussion of study results include all issues of concern to users?

Data from Refs.[10,11,15–22]

in each study listed in descending order. Fracture fixation, either by open reduction and internal fixation or by external fixation, was the most common type of procedure performed in 5 out of the 7 studies that provided breakdown of procedure types. Other common procedures included wound debridement, amputation, and contracture release. It should be noted that Grimes and colleagues[17] performed 1063 manipulations under anesthesia. Although this is not considered a surgery, the authors included it as a type of procedure. Each of the 10 studies featured outreach efforts that operated on all bones and joints featured in general orthopedic surgery, with the notable exception of Tadisina and colleagues[11] who focused solely on pathology of the hand and forearm.

Degree of Cost-Effectiveness

All 10 studies used the cost per DALY averted as the cost-effectiveness. The degree of cost-effectiveness ranged from $10.70 per DALY averted for Roberts and colleagues[19] providing

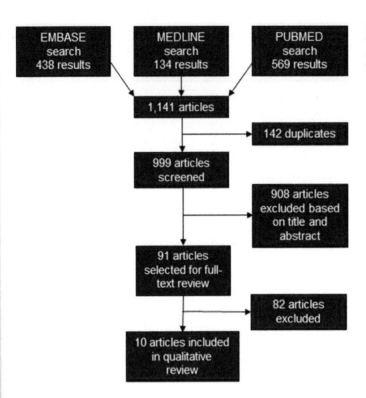

Fig. 1. PRISMA diagram documenting the search strategy results and final records included in this qualitative systematic review.

orthopedic and obstetric care through a nongovernmental organization in Zambia to $532.11 per DALY averted for Gosselin and colleagues[15] comparing elective versus emergent orthopedic

outreach in the Dominican Republic and Nicaragua. Threshold values for cost-effectiveness, in accordance with the WHO-CHOICE guidelines, are presented in **Table 7** for LMICs in the studies

Table 4
Brief summary of outreach effort for included studies

Author, Year	Brief Summary of Outreach Effort
Carlson et al,[18] 2012	Two-year orthopedic trauma specialist training program for doctors in Haiti
Chen et al,[16] 2012	Volunteer team providing orthopedic surgical care for 30 patients at a Nicaraguan hospital
Gosselin et al,[20] 2006	Nongovernmental organization–run hospital providing trauma care to victims injured by war in Sierra Leone
Gosselin & Heitto,[10] 2008	Nongovernmental organization–run hospital providing trauma care to victims injured by war in Cambodia
Gosselin et al,[21] 2010	Volunteer team providing trauma care at 2 Medecins Sans Frontieres hospitals in Nigeria and Haiti
Gosselin et al,[15] 2011	Comparative analysis of providing orthopedic care in the elective vs emergent setting
Grimes et al,[17,34] 2014	Training of orthopedic clinical providers in Malawi
Rattray et al,[22] 2013	Volunteer outreach through a multidisciplinary surgical center for children in Cambodia
Roberts et al,[19] 2016	Providing orthopedic and obstetric care through a nongovernmental organization in Zambia
Tadisina et al,[11] 2014	Visiting surgeons performing hand surgery in Honduras for 1 wk

Data from Refs.[10,11,15–22]

Table 5
Summary of outreach efforts and cost-effectiveness for included studies

Author, Year	Location	Length	Type of Surgery	Elective vs. Emergent	Trauma Focused	Attempt to Establish Infrastructure	Unit of Cost-Effectiveness Outcome	Cost per Outcome (2016 USD)
Carlson et al,[18] 2012	Haiti	2 y	Orthopedic	Elective	Yes	Yes	$ per DALY averted	$36.28
Chen et al,[16] 2012	Nicaragua	1 wk	Orthopedic	Elective	No	No	$ per DALY averted	$378.44
Gosselin et al,[20] 2006	Sierra Leone	3 mo	General, orthopedic	Elective	Yes	Yes	$ per DALY averted	$39.30
Gosselin & Heitto,[10] 2008	Cambodia	3 mo	General, orthopedic	Elective	Yes	Yes	$ per DALY averted	$85.61
Gosselin et al,[21] 2010	Haiti, Nigeria	3 mo	General, orthopedic	Elective	Yes	Yes	$ per DALY averted	$193.11
Gosselin et al,[15] 2011	Dominican Republic, Nicaragua	8 wk	Orthopedic	Both	Yes	No	$ per DALY averted	$532.11
Grimes et al,[17,34] 2014	Malawi	3 wk	Orthopedic	Elective	Yes	Yes	$ per DALY averted	$93.24
Rattray et al,[22] 2013	Cambodia	2 mo	Ophthalmologic, orthopedic, plastic reconstructive	Elective	No	Yes	$ per DALY averted	$101.85
Roberts et al,[19] 2016	Zambia	2 mo	Obstetric, orthopedic	Both	No	Yes	$ per DALY averted	$10.70
Tadisina et al,[11] 2014	Honduras	1 wk	Orthopedic	Elective	No	No	$ per DALY averted	$524.95

Data from Refs.[10,11,15–22]

Table 6
Total and most common orthopedic procedures performed by study[a]

Author, Year	Total Orthopedic Procedures	Most Common Procedure (% of Total)	Second Most Common Procedure (% of Total)	Third Most Common Procedure (% of Total)
Gosselin et al,[20] 2006	N = 338	Fracture fixation (33%)	Wound debridement (21%)	Burn debridement/ repair (13%)
Gosselin & Heitto,[10] 2008	N = 753	Fracture fixation (46%)	Wound debridement (39%)	Contracture release (6%)
Gosselin et al,[15] 2011	N = 253	Fracture fixation (28%)	Wound debridement (22%)	Congenital malformation repair (16%)
Grimes et al,[17,34] 2014	N = 1313	Manipulation under anesthesia (81%)	Fracture fixation (16%)	Amputation (2%)
Rattray et al,[22] 2013	N = 34	Fracture fixation (55%)	Arthroscopy (17%)	Arthroplasty (13%)
Roberts et al,[19] 2016	N = 155	Fracture fixation (85%)	Amputation (14%)	Not provided
Tadisina et al,[11] 2014	N = 128	Contracture release (17%)	Fracture fixation and/or tendon repair (15%)	Congenital malformation repair (14%)

[a] Chen et al. (2012) and Gosselin et al. (2010) did not provide a breakdown of orthopedic procedure type and was therefore not included in this chart.
Data from Refs.[10,11,15–22]

meeting criteria for this review. Based on these thresholds, all included studies presented interventions that are very cost-effective.

DISCUSSION

The findings of this review strongly suggest that providing orthopedic surgical interventions in LMICs can be very cost-effective. Although

Table 7
Cost-effectiveness threshold levels, as defined by WHO-CHOICE, for low- and middle-income countries featured in this review

Country	Threshold Level	
	2016 Per-Capita GDP	2016 Per-Capita GDP x 3
Cambodia	$1228	$3684
Dominican Republic	$7083	$21,249
Haiti	$761	$2283
Honduras	$2551	$7653
Malawi	$294	$882
Nicaragua	$2115	$6345
Nigeria	$2260	$6780
Sierra Leone	$666	$1998
Zambia	$1231	$3693

this was true regardless of location, emergent versus nonemergent surgery, and traumatic versus nontraumatic pathology, certain intervention types may be relatively more cost-effective than others. For example, Gosselin and colleagues[15] compared providing care in elective versus relief situations in Central America and the Caribbean, finding that interventions in relief situations were slightly more cost-effective ($343 per DALY averted) than those in elective situations ($362). Similarly, Roberts and colleagues provided both orthopedic and obstetric surgeries in a relief setting with the greatest cost-effectiveness of all studies included in this review ($10.70 per DALY averted).[19] Although the latter result may be partly attributable to the obstetric care provided, a traditionally highly cost-effective specialty in LMICs, one cannot underestimate the role of volunteering in a relief situation. And despite the belief that the less-organized environment of a relief setting may lead to inefficiency and poor allocation of resources, the novel and tremendous volume of patients with considerable long-term disability may drive the potential for superior cost-effectiveness.

In regard to interventions for traumatic versus nontraumatic conditions, there is undoubtedly a greater burden of disease in LMICs for posttraumatic states. However, these findings suggest not only that there is a greater need for traumatic interventions but also that these interventions may result in superior cost-effectiveness compared with nontraumatic issues. For example, Carlson and colleagues[18] and the 2006 study by Gosselin and colleagues[20] reported the second and third greatest overall cost-effectiveness, respectively, in the authors' review, both of which having focused primarily on trauma surgery. In fact, more than one-third of the procedures performed by Gosselin and colleagues were open reduction and internal fixations, closely followed by wound debridement and burn repair. The high incidence of trauma in LMICs, combined with the effectiveness and relative commonality of procedures such as these, can result in considerable cost-effectiveness.

Outreach efforts aimed at sustainability were also particularly cost-effective. Studies that documented efforts to establish or contribute to local infrastructure were more cost-effective (mean of $80.01 per DALY averted) than efforts that did not necessarily attempt to establish infrastructure (mean of $478.50 per DALY averted).[10,17–22] Although contributions to local infrastructure can result in sizable long-term economic benefit, the disparity in these numbers is likely due to several additional factors. Firstly, the immediate cost of setting up a temporary clinic or surgical setting for a 1-week outreach effort is considerable, especially if the site is to be dismantled on completion of the trip rather than continue to be used by local providers. Secondly, several of the studies that contributed to infrastructure represented outreach efforts at established hospital systems in LMICs. These established hospital systems may have preformed routines for clinical assessment and surgery, greater familiarity with the language and culture of the patient population, and providers with specialized roles that do not have to travel with the volunteer team. Each of these can contribute to a more efficient outreach effort.

The ultimate embodiment of establishing infrastructure is through the training of local orthopedic providers. Although many studies contain some aspect of inherent training or instruction, few perform economic analysis of the educative efforts. However, both Carlson and colleagues[18] and Grimes and colleagues[17] analyzed the cost-effectiveness of an education through training programs for orthopedic specialists in Haiti and Malawi, respectively, realizing a cost-effectiveness of $36.28 and $93.24 per DALY. This type of analysis is unique in that it estimates the value of surgeries provided for years to come following the conclusion of the education. Although this form of outreach carries new challenges, educative efforts have the potential to be extremely cost-effective and have been supported by some as the most feasible solutions to the global shortage of surgical care.[23,24]

The growing need for surgical care in the developing world is not unique to orthopedic surgery, and there has been a growing focus on publicizing outreach efforts across all fields of medicine. Although not all outreach efforts in LMICs can claim to be cost-effective by WHO CHOICE standards,[9,25] several recent studies have highlighted surgical subspecialties other than orthopedics that may provide cost-effective care. These include cataract removal (cost per DALY averted $5–106 USD),[26–28] circumcision and hernia repair (cost/DALY averted $7–320 USD),[29–31] maternal obstetric care (cost per DALY averted $18–3420 USD),[7,32] and cleft lip and palate repair (cost per DALY averted $15–96 USD).[33,34] With a range of $10.70 to $532.11 per DALY averted, this review suggests that the cost-effectiveness of orthopedic interventions is comparable to other types of surgical care. Similarly, these data compare favorably to medical public health interventions such as oral rehydration therapy ($1062 per DALY averted), breast feeding promotion ($930 per DALY averted), and highly active antiretroviral therapy for human immunodeficiency virus ($922 per DALY averted).[2,34,35]

This study is not without limitations. As for any systematic review, slight publication bias is inevitable. However, the authors emphasize on the different characteristics that made certain interventions more cost-effective. In addition, the studies examined in this systematic review did not adhere to the same methodology to calculate cost-effectiveness. The quality of the articles included in the final analysis was examined using the Drummond checklist and found that for the 10 articles included in the analysis, the quality of each study was generally uniform. Furthermore, the main objective was not to determine the overall cost-effectiveness for orthopedic surgery in the developing world. Rather, it was to determine whether individual interventions were cost-effective according to WHO-CHOICE methods and to analyze the different characteristics of these interventions.

SUMMARY

Injuries and musculoskeletal disorders are key contributors to the global burden of disease, with a disproportionately high burden on those living in the developing world. This review of the literature found that outreach efforts focused on addressing this need through orthopedic surgery have been universally very cost-effective according to WHO-CHOICE thresholds. This was especially true for efforts that focused on providing trauma-related care, functioned in relief situations, or aimed to contribute to local sustainability of care. In addition, the cost-effectiveness of orthopedic outreach efforts compare favorably to both other surgical specialties and medical public health interventions. These results should be encouraging for both orthopedic surgeons planning outreach efforts and organizers and donators who are considering providing funds and other resources to orthopedic outreach. Allocation of appropriate resources can help alleviate a major burden of disease and improve quality of life for individuals living in LMICs.

REFERENCES

1. World Health Organization. The global burden of disease: annex A: deaths and DALYs 2004 annex tables. In: WHO, editor. The global burden of disease. Geneva (Switzerland): World Health Organization; 2004.

2. Bickler SN, Weiser TG, Kassebaum N, et al. Global burden of surgical conditions. In: Debas HT, Donkor P, Gawande A, et al, editors. Essential surgery: disease control priorities, third edition, vol. 1. Washington, DC: The International Bank for Reconstruction and Development/The World Bank; 2015. p. 19–40.

3. Alkire BC, Shrime MG, Dare AJ, et al. Global economic consequences of selected surgical diseases: a modelling study. Lancet Glob Health 2015;3(Suppl 2):S21–7.

4. Chung KY. Plastic and reconstructive surgery in global health: let's reconstruct global surgery. Plast Reconstr Surg Glob Open 2017;5(4):e1273.

5. Dieleman JL, Graves C, Johnson E, et al. Sources and focus of health development assistance, 1990-2014. JAMA 2015;313(23):2359–68.

6. Evans DB, Adam T, Edejer TT, et al. Time to reassess strategies for improving health in developing countries. BMJ 2005;331(7525):1133–6.

7. Alkire BC, Vincent JR, Burns CT, et al. Obstructed labor and caesarean delivery: the cost and benefit of surgical intervention. PLoS One 2012;7(4):e34595.

8. Wittenborn JS, Rein DB. Cost-effectiveness of glaucoma interventions in Barbados and Ghana. Optom Vis Sci 2011;88(1):155–63.

9. Zelle SG, Nyarko KM, Bosu WK, et al. Costs, effects and cost-effectiveness of breast cancer control in Ghana. Trop Med Int Health 2012;17(8):1031–43.

10. Gosselin RA, Heitto M. Cost-effectiveness of a district trauma hospital in Battambang, Cambodia. World J Surg 2008;32(11):2450–3.

11. Tadisina KK, Chopra K, Tangredi J, et al. Helping hands: a cost-effectiveness study of a humanitarian hand surgery mission. Plast Surg Int 2014;2014:921625.

12. Moher D, Liberati A, Tetzlaff J, et al. Preferred reporting items for systematic reviews and meta-analyses: the PRISMA statement. Ann Intern Med 2009;151(4):264–9. w264.

13. World Health Organization. Prevention CfDCa. International classification of diseases, tenth revision, clinical modification (ICD-10-CM) 2017. Geneva (Switzerland): World Health Organization; 2017. Available at: https://icd.who.int/browse10/2016/en.

14. Drummond ME, Sculpher MJ, Torrance GW, et al. Methods for the economic evaluation of health care programmes. 3rd edition. New York: Oxford medical publications; 2005.

15. Gosselin RA, Gialamas G, Atkin DM. Comparing the cost-effectiveness of short orthopedic missions in elective and relief situations in developing countries. World J Surg 2011;35(5):951–5.

16. Chen AT, Pedtke A, Kobs JK, et al. Volunteer orthopedic surgical trips in Nicaragua: a cost-effectiveness evaluation. World J Surg 2012;36(12):2802–8.

17. Grimes CE, Mkandawire NC, Billingsley ML, et al. The cost-effectiveness of orthopaedic clinical officers in Malawi. Trop Doct 2014;44(3):128–34.

18. Carlson LC, Slobogean GP, Pollak AN. Orthopaedic trauma care in Haiti: a cost-effectiveness analysis of an innovative surgical residency program. Value Health 2012;15(6):887–93.

19. Roberts G, Roberts C, Jamieson A, et al. Surgery and obstetric care are highly cost-effective interventions in a sub-saharan african district hospital: a three-month single-institution study of surgical costs and outcomes. World J Surg 2016;40(1):14–20.

20. Gosselin RA, Thind A, Bellardinelli A. Cost/DALY averted in a small hospital in Sierra Leone: what is the relative contribution of different services? World J Surg 2006;30(4):505–11.

21. Gosselin RA, Maldonado A, Elder G. Comparative cost-effectiveness analysis of two MSF surgical trauma centers. World J Surg 2010;34(3):415–9.

22. Rattray KW, Harrop Tara C, Aird J, et al. The cost effectiveness of reconstructive surgery in Cambodia. Asian Biomed 2013;7:319.

23. Riviello R, Ozgediz D, Hsia RY, et al. Role of collaborative academic partnerships in surgical training, education, and provision. World J Surg 2010;34(3):459–65.

24. Mitchell KB, Giiti G, Kotecha V, et al. Surgical education at Weill Bugando Medical Centre: supplementing surgical training and investing in local health care providers. Can J Surg 2013;56(3):199–203.

25. Horton S, Gelband H, Jamison D, et al. Ranking 93 health interventions for low- and middle-income countries by cost-effectiveness. PLoS One 2017;12(8):e0182951.

26. Singh AJ, Garner P, Floyd K. Cost-effectiveness of public-funded options for cataract surgery in Mysore, India. Lancet 2000;355(9199):180–4.

27. Marseille E. Cost-effectiveness of cataract surgery in a public health eye care programme in Nepal. Bull World Health Organ 1996;74(3):319–24.

28. Baltussen R, Sylla M, Mariotti SP. Cost-effectiveness analysis of cataract surgery: a global and regional analysis. Bull World Health Organ 2004;82(5):338–45.

29. Binagwaho A, Pegurri E, Muita J, et al. Male circumcision at different ages in Rwanda: a cost-effectiveness study. PLoS Med 2010;7(1):e1000211.

30. Bollinger LA, Stover J, Musuka G, et al. The cost and impact of male circumcision on HIV/AIDS in Botswana. J Int AIDS Soc 2009;12:7.

31. Shillcutt SD, Sanders DL, Teresa Butron-Vila M, et al. Cost-effectiveness of inguinal hernia surgery in northwestern Ecuador. World J Surg 2013;37(1):32–41.

32. Adam T, Lim SS, Mehta S, et al. Cost effectiveness analysis of strategies for maternal and neonatal health in developing countries. BMJ 2005;331(7525):1107.

33. Alkire B, Hughes CD, Nash K, et al. Potential economic benefit of cleft lip and palate repair in sub-Saharan Africa. World J Surg 2011;35(6):1194–201.

34. Grimes CE, Henry JA, Maraka J, et al. Cost-effectiveness of surgery in low- and middle-income countries: a systematic review. World J Surg 2014;38(1):252–63.

35. Meara JG, Leather AJ, Hagander L, et al. Global Surgery 2030: evidence and solutions for achieving health, welfare, and economic development. Lancet 2015;386(9993):569–624.

Global Hand Surgery
Initiatives that Work (The Touching Hands Project): Why, When, and How!

Scott H. Kozin, MD[a,b,c,d,*]

KEYWORDS

- Touching Hands Project • Global hand surgery • Volunteerism • Outreach
- American Foundation for Surgery of the Hand • American Society for Surgery of the Hand

KEY POINTS

- The Touching Hands Project was initiated as part of the American Society for Surgery of the Hand (ASSH) outreach effort in 2014.
- The project has expanded rapidly and has become a pillar along with education, research, clinical practice (patient care), and organizational excellence.
- The Touching Hands Project in collaboration with organizations with similar missions has greatly expanded hand care across the globe by focusing on education, patient care, surgery, and rehabilitation.

INTRODUCTION INTO AMERICAN SOCIETY FOR SURGERY OF THE HAND

The American Society for Surgery of the Hand (ASSH) was started shortly after World War II by 3 great Americans: a politician (Franklin Delano Roosevelt), a general (Norman T. Kirk), and an innovative surgeon (Sterling Bunnell).[1] All 3 men were early twentieth century Americans and important men in the genesis of the hand surgery. Franklin Delano Roosevelt overcame the devastation of poliomyelitis to become President of the United States. Norman T. Kirk was an army surgeon for 35 years. His specialty transitioned from general surgery to orthopedic surgery based on his experiences with amputees from World War I. Dr Kirk became Chief Surgeon at Letterman Hospital in San Francisco. There he met Sterling Bunnell, the father of hand surgery. Sterling Bunnell had served in France in the US

Army. He was prolific in performing research, operating, and publishing on every topic in hand surgery. Both Bunnell and Kirk were avid hunters and anglers, and their friendship blossomed. Roosevelt navigated the Unites States through World War II and desired to do more for the returning injured soldiers. The Commander-in-Chief appointed orthopedic surgeon Norman T. Kirk to the post of Surgeon General of the Army. He was appalled at the number of "crippled hands" he found in the 78 hospitals around the United States that cared for our injured soldiers. He immediately asked Bunnell for help, which prompted Bunnell to close his office for 2 years at the age of 62. Bunnell established Centers for Hand Surgery and personally selected the surgeons to direct them. He felt strongly that a single specialized surgeon should provide comprehensive care to the hand, including skin, tendon, nerve, vasculature, and

Disclosure: The author has nothing to disclose.
[a] Touching Hands Project, ASSH, Chicago, IL, USA; [b] Shriners Hospitals for Children–Philadelphia, 3551 North Broad Street, Philadelphia, PA 19140, USA; [c] Lewis Katz School of Medicine, Temple University School of Medicine, Philadelphia, PA, USA; [d] Sidney Kimmel Medical College of Thomas Jefferson University, Philadelphia, PA, USA
* Shriners Hospitals for Children–Philadelphia, 3551 North Broad Street, Philadelphia, PA 19140.
E-mail address: skozin@shrinenet.org

bones. These Hand Centers cared for more than 10,000 patients before closure long after the war had ended. This group of ingenious and dedicated individuals paved the way for the ASSH. Their first meeting was held in 1946 with Sterling Bunnell as the first president.

GROWTH: MEMBERSHIP, OFFICE, WEALTH

The ASSH expanded over the next 50 years with a focus on patient care, education, and research. In 1998, the central office moved from Denver, Colorado to Chicago, Illinois. The ASSH financial situation contained about $1 million in operations and $2 million in research money via the American Foundation for Surgery of the Hand (AFSH), established in 1987. Mark Anderson, CAE became the Chief Executive Officer with lofty goals for the organization to truly become the world leader and authority in hand surgery. The current mission statement (2014) reads that the ASSH will advance the science and practice of hand and upper-extremity surgery through education, research, and advocacy on behalf of patients and practitioners. The vision statement states that the ASSH will be recognized as the most reliable and authoritative source of information on all aspects of hand and upper-extremity disorders for all audiences, surgeons, allied health professionals, government, business and industry, patients, and the public.

The ASSH leadership realized that to fulfill the mission and obtain the vision, resources were necessary to succeed. From 1998 through 2012, the ASSH central office resided within the Academy of Orthopaedic Surgeons office building. During this time, the ASSH continued to evolve, mature, and expand the services offered to the members, patients, and researchers. The ASSH financial holdings grew to $15 million in operations and $7 million in research money via the AFSH.

In 2012, the ASSH leadership made the bold decision to purchase a freestanding building in the West Loop of Chicago. The leadership of ASSH expanded opportunities for members, enhanced membership benefits, and developed new programs. The calculated approach and herculean effort resulted in the ASSH becoming the world leader in hand surgery, the authority in hand surgery, and fulfillment of the vision started by Sterling Bunnell. The current coffers total approximately $20 million for ASSH and nearly $20 million for the AFSH: a truly remarkable growth attributed to dedicated leadership, hardworking central office, and tremendous membership support.

PRESIDENTIAL LINE INITIATIVES/AMERICAN SOCIETY FOR SURGERY OF THE HAND PILLARS

In 2010, the presidential line of the ASSH decided that "presidential" initiatives should be transformed into presidential line initiatives. Presidential initiatives often prospered during the president's term and frequently floundered afterward. Presidential line initiatives stood the test of time and were implemented into the ethos of the ASSH. This simple change in governance resulted in remarkable projects that lasted well beyond the tenure of the presidential line. Presidential line initiatives included purchasing an independent building, launching an on-line platform for education (Hand-E), publishing a Hand Society Textbook, and establishing outreach (Touching Hands Project, http://www.assh.org/touching-hands).

After the launching of The Touching Hands Project, the presidential line and council members (task force) convened to assess the "pillars" of the hand society. Education, research, and patient care had dominated the efforts of the Hand Society. The task force proposed that 2 additional pillars be added to the mission of the ASSH. The first was organizational excellence. The central office has been the core the ASSH's success with talented hardworking individuals dedicated to improve the society. Their diligence has been an integral part of the overall success of the organization. The second pillar was outreach, including international and domestic efforts to "provide life-changing hand surgeries, rehabilitation, and medical training in the world's poorest communities" (Fig. 1).

AMERICAN SOCIETY FOR SURGERY OF THE HAND PRESIDENCY 2014 (68TH PRESIDENT OF THE AMERICAN SOCIETY FOR SURGERY OF THE HAND)

My presidential address to the members the ASSH (2014) discussed the growth and prosperity of the organization since its inception in 1946.[2] I discussed the roots of the organization and the pioneers of hand surgery, including Paul Brand, MD. Dr Brand devoted his career to persons less fortunate and was the consummate altruistic physician missionary. He dispelled many of the misperceptions regarding leprosy patients, also known as the untouchables. His accomplishments are detailed in the book entitled, *The Gift of Pain*, authored by Dr Brand and Philip Yancey.[3] For example, there was a

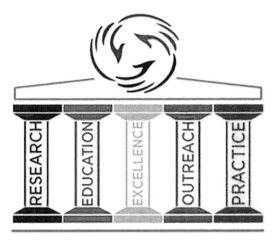

American Society for
Surgery of the Hand

Fig. 1. Pillar of the ASSH. (*Courtesy of* American Society for Surgery of the Hand, Chicago, IL.)

common belief that, in patients afflicted with leprosy, their fingers and toes fell off secondary to the "bad flesh" of leprosy. Dr Brand doubted this concept and lived with the untouchables to assess their daily life. He established sentinels to stay up all night and observe the patients sleeping. One night, a rat climbed onto the bed of a patient, sniffed around the person's hand, nuzzled a finger, met no resistance, and subsequently gnawed on the finger, biting away the flesh. Because leprosy results in the loss of feeling, the patient slept soundly, unaware of the rat causing digital destruction. Dr Brand emphasized the necessity of afferent pain signals to negate harm to our extremities, in both our feet and our hands.

My address emphasized the compassion of contemporary mentors and leaders in the ASSH, such as Peter Stern, MD. Dr Stern provided the Founder's lecture in 2013 and addressed the membership with his lecture entitled, "Far from the Bedside." He stated that "volunteerism is the essence of clinical medicine—you truly make a difference in people's lives. The appeal of these trips comes from making new friends from a different culture, having the opportunity to teach third-world health care professionals who are starving for medical knowledge, and you perform challenging surgeries in suboptimal conditions necessitating creativity and innovation." My address quoted Peter Carter, MD, who spoke to the incoming American Academy of Orthopaedic Surgeons in 2005, professing, "earning a living is important, and sometimes even interesting—but

sooner or later...making a difference is what counts. I encourage all of you to find some time to do what you do best for someone who really needs it, and then give it away. You will be repaid in ways you cannot begin to expect."

My address detailed the meteoric rise of the Hand Society regarding growth (membership, monies, and prestige). I challenged the membership to do more for humanity, to expand hand care to the "have nots" in this world. I further stated that the world is not a fair place, with one-half of the world living on less than $2 per day. I quoted Martin Luther King Jr, who stated, "of all the forms of inequity, injustice in health is the most shocking and the most inhumane."

I concluded with a metaphor emphasizing that the world is like a cleft hand with a large divide between those who have access to hand care and those who do not have access to hand care. I stated that we (the ASSH) are the surgeons who can close the cleft and fix the divide via The Touching Hands Project. In addition, it is our duty and social obligation as leaders in health care to participate in outreach for humanity. Service is part of the ethos of the ASSH just waiting to be harnessed more effectively. I ended with on a last quote from Albert Pine, an English author circa 1850: "What we do for ourselves dies with us. What we do for others and the world remains and is immortal."

TOUCHING HANDS PROJECT, INAUGURAL MISSION, 2014

The inaugural Touching Hands Mission occurred in 2014. A group of 11 committed health care professionals (surgeons, anesthesiologists, therapists) traveled to Haiti, the poorest country in the northern hemisphere (**Fig. 2**). The poverty was overwhelming; the poorness was unthinkable, and the living conditions were deplorable. The earthquake of 2010 shattered a tenuous living situation. The chronic poverty and despair were unable to withstand the acute earthquake and all its devastation.

The Touching Hands mission performed evaluations and surgeries at the Haiti Adventist Hospital, located in the midst of the Port au Prince poverty. Fittingly, the hospital motto reads, "Plant a seed you reap a tree, teach someone to plant a tree you reap a forest." The city was abounding with tent camps, stray dogs, and poor people. The air was filled with the odor of open fires and the stink of spoiled trash.

The hospital had makeshift operating rooms, and supplies were scarce; however, The Touching Hands team carried 700 pounds of supplies with

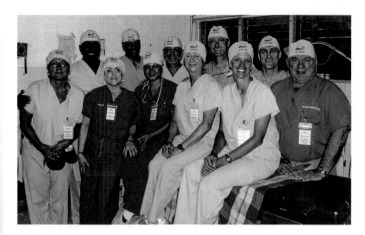

Fig. 2. Inaugural touching hands mission to Haiti team members (*front row, left to right*: Kim Russo, CRNA, Susan Shappiro, RN, Sophorn Mot, CRNA, Christine Novak, OTR/L, Rebecca von der Heyde, OTR/L; *back row, left to right*: Garvey Jonassaint, RN, George Dyer, MD, Scott Kozin, MD, Mark Baratz, MD, Mike Nakashian, MD, Harry Bonet, MD).

them, many donated by corporate sponsors. The Touching Hands team speedily got to work. We evaluated patients with familiar and unfamiliar conditions, many with injuries related to the earthquake. We assembled an operating list of patients, giving priority to those in most need. We brought headlights because the power grid was notoriously unstable, and frequently the lights turned off during the procedure.

The week was full of clinic patients and surgical cases.

The Touching Hands team bonded and overcame the obstacles of limited supplies, poor lighting, and an overabundance of patients. The team was on a mission to Haiti, and no hardship was going to stop us from caring. The Haitians were struggling to overcome a 7.0 earthquake, and the least we could do was to overcome lack of lighting or insufficient hardware.

As the team traveled back to the United States, we realized that this effort was going to require time and money for the hand care and education necessary in Haiti. The Touching Hand Project must be committed to provide the necessary surgical expertise, education, and support to help the Haitian people. Hand surgery and rehabilitation could restore hand function and give the Haitians the ability to work with their hands so they can improve their dire situation and lessen their entrenched poverty.

LANCET COMMISSION 2014

Global health initiatives focused on vaccination programs, malaria control, parasite management, and medications to treat diseases. Surgical global health received minimal attention regarding its effectiveness and needed financial support. The concept that global surgery was marginally effective changed dramatically in 2014 when *The*

Lancet commission published a timely position statement on surgical care and global health.[4] The commission found there were gross disparities in access to safe and essential surgical care worldwide. There was also an alarming lack of global focus on quality surgical services. Modest estimates showed that at least 2 billion people worldwide lacked access to basic surgical care. Approximately 250 million operations are performed each year with only 3.5% performed on the poorest one-third of the world's population. Low-income and middle-income countries bear the greatest burden of untreated surgical disease.

Furthermore, an estimated 11% to 15% of the world's disability is secondary to surgically treatable conditions. Injuries alone cause 5.7 million deaths per year, far greater than the 3.8 million deaths caused by malaria, human immunodeficiency virus (HIV)/AIDS, and tuberculosis combined. Surgical treatment was identified as a cost-effective intervention in resource-poor settings, equal to vaccination programs and 10 to 15 times more effective than antiretroviral medication for HIV.

The commission stated that this discrepancy in surgical care was a moral imperative to address the inequities in global surgery. The commission was not claiming surgery was any more important than other types of treatment; however, it is certainly on par with other global health priorities. The commission elevated the role and importance of global surgery by propelling The Touching Hands Project into the mainstream.

TOUCHING HANDS PROJECT, MENTORSHIP AND GUIDANCE, 2014

The ASSH leadership and The Touching Hands Project contributors quickly realized that mentorship and guidance were necessary for success.

The group reached out to Bill Magee, MD, who founded Operation Smile in 1982. The organization is the standard-bearer nongovernmental organization (NGO) that provides cleft lip and palate repair surgeries to children worldwide. Operation Smile has a multifaceted approach to cleft lip and palate, including developing ambassadorships to raise awareness of cleft issues, sponsoring a world care program for international cases requiring specialized care, and organizing articles and foundations worldwide to assist countries in reaching self-sufficiency with cleft surgeries. Operation Smile has provided hundreds of thousands of free surgeries for children and young adults born with cleft lips, cleft palates, and other facial deformities in more than 60 countries since its inception.

A small ASSH group traveled to Operation Smile's headquarters in Norfolk, Virginia in 2014 (**Fig. 3**). The goal was to seek guidance and mentorship from Bill Magee and his team. We spent the day meeting with various integral members of Operation Smile and learning from each of them. We sought advice to each part of their operation's team, including mission organization, supply coordination, financial development, donor recognition, and more.

The visit was memorable and directed The Touching Hands Project toward a pathway of success. Bill Magee has remained a supporter of the ASSH and The Touching Hands Project. His sage advice and ongoing input continue to be invaluable.

COLLABORATION

Following a single successful mission in 2014, The Touching Hands Project explored methods to expand to more sites, which offered more opportunity for ASSH members to participate. One successful approach has been collaboration with organizations that possess similar missions and visions. This collaborative effort has resulted in combined missions with other NGOs, such as Resurge International (Bolivia, Vietnam, Cambodia), Guatemala Healing Hands (Guatemala), Cure Hospital (Ethiopia), and World Pediatric Project (St. Vincent and the Grenadines). James Chang, MD was the 72nd president of the ASSH and is the Chief Medical Officer of Resurge International and fostered the symbiotic relationship between The Touching Hands Project and Resurge. These collaborative efforts between similar organizations have been mutually beneficial. The Touching Hands Project provides mission participants with hand surgical and rehabilitation expertise. In addition, the mission members bring supplies that are donated and/or unavailable in-country.

Concurrently, The Touching Hands Project has continued to develop independent missions with countries or organizations interested in partnering with The Touching Hands Project. This effort has led to established missions in Trinidad and Tobago (Caribbean Health Foundation) and Honduras (Ruth Paz Clinic) (**Fig. 4**).

The Touching Hands Project also realized that many members participated in independent

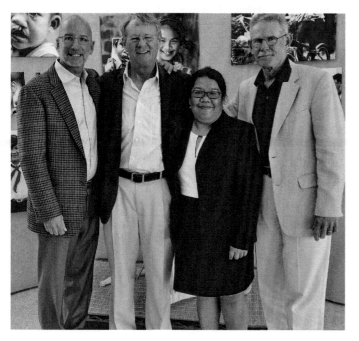

Fig. 3. Representatives of the ASSH visited Operation Smile's headquarters in Norfolk, Virginia in 2014 (Scott Kozin, MD, William Magee, MD, Angie Legaspi, CMP, William Seitz, MD).

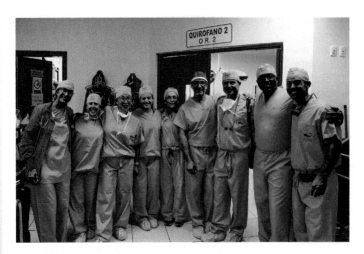

Fig. 4. Members of The Touching Hand Project in Honduras working in collaboration with the Ruth Paz Clinic (Marcy Tucker, MD, Jennifer Hertz, MD, Jeanette Lee, MD, Chelsea Leversedge, BS, Sue Shapiro, RN, Scott Kozin, MD, Fraser Leversedge, MD, Garvey Jonassaint, RN, Jeremy Miles, MD).

missions with other organization that were equally worthwhile. As the donations and funding grew, The Touching Hands Project offered funds to help support those members' travel and expenses. Members have completed missions to numerous countries, including Vietnam, Rwanda, Guatemala, Dominican Republican, Nepal, Burkina Faso, and Peru.

CORPORATE SOCIAL RESPONSIBILITY/ SUPPLIES

Corporate social responsibility is a buzzword that is synonymous with corporate sustainability, sustainable business, corporate conscience, corporate citizenship, and conscious capitalism.

Although the term is controversial with respect to intention, ethical ideologies, and motive, The Touching Hands Project has reaped the benefits of corporate social responsibility. Industry partners that are firm believers in corporate social responsibility have provided financial support and donated invaluable amounts of medical supplies to The Touching Hands Project. The list of Touching Hands Project partners is impressive (**Table 1**).

The partners can donate supplies, sponsor a mission, or make a financial donation. Sponsoring an entire mission has the added benefit of sending a representative. Stryker has been the largest sponsor of entire missions and has sent employees to Haiti and Honduras. Todd Schrader, senior director of Marketing at Stryker, accompanied The Touching Hands team to Haiti in 2015. Todd stated, "This was a life changer for me. I was truly humbled by the selflessness of the entire team of

Table 1
The Touching Hands Project partners

Americares	Esperanca, Inc	Lee Gordon Fund
Axogen, Inc	Ethicon	MAP International
Baxter/Tissel	Fundación Ruth Paz	Medartis
The Bonet Family	GOJO Industries	
Hospital Sisters Health System	Guatemala Healing Hands Foundation	Hand Surgery Endowment
CURE International	Checkpoint Surgical	OHK Medical Devices
DePuy Synthes	Integra Foundation	
	Shriners Hospitals for Children	Medtronic Musculoskeletal Transplant Foundation
Johnson & Johnson	Purell	Duke University
ReSurge International	OrthoPediatrics	SanMar
Stryker	TriMed	Zimmer Biomet
Wright Medical Technology	World Pediatric Project	

healthcare professionals that were on the trip. For me, it is clear that everyone, not just the healthcare professionals, can play a role and contribute." These words echo those of other volunteers who have been similarly affected by the experience of participating in a Touching Hands mission.

The influx of donations and the management of supplies necessitated the appointment of Susan Shapiro, RN as volunteer supply coordinator (Manager of Medical Missions Supply Services) for The Touching Hands Project. Susan dedicates an inordinate amount of time and effort to ensure the mission has ample equipment and supplies to succeed. The necessary items vary tremendously from drapes/gowns/gloves to drills/plates/screws to intravenous tubing/syringes/anesthetic medications. The overall list is impressive, and the herculean task is currently delegated to a single volunteer. The Touching Hands Project is looking at avenues to coordinate and streamline the process.

DOMESTIC MISSIONS

The concept of providing free care to those underinsured or uninsured in the United Sates was always complicated by licensure and liability. Initially, these were insurmountable obstacles. In 2016, John Seiler, MD, while serving as AFSH president, singlehandedly overcame these hurdles and started domestic outreach. He used local hand surgeons who already had licensure and liability coverage in a surgery center that donated their building and ancillaries to the community outreach effort.

The first domestic hand day occurred in Atlanta, Georgia under the leadership of John Seiler, MD and Houston Payne, MD. Volunteers included surgeons (attendings, fellows, residents), nurses, anesthesiologists, and paramedical personnel devoted to caring. This model has been expanded year after year, including additional cities, such as Nashville, Tennessee; Philadelphia, Pennsylvania; Salt Lake City, Utah; Dayton, Ohio; and more. Volunteers can provide free care and treatment in a single day without the expense and burden of weeklong international mission work.

ENDOWMENT

The ASSH and the AFSH embraced the importance of outreach and The Touching Hands Project. The leaderships decided to raise substantial monies and form an endowment for outreach. The lofty goal of $5 million was established (go big or go home!). Leaders from the ASSH included Mark Anderson, CAE, William Seitz, MD, Neil Jones, MD, Ghazi Rayan, MD, and James Chang, MD. AFSH leaders included John Bednar, MD, John Seiler, MD, Steven Glickel, MD, and Terry Light, MD.

During James Chang's, MD presidency in 2018, the $5 million goal was reached! In just 4 years, The Touching Hands Project was endowed in perpetuity. The outreach pillar was firmly established in character and funding. Outreach and The Touching Hands Project assumed the added responsibility as stewards of the endowment, ensuring that spending aligns with the mission and fulfills the vision of The Touching Hands Project.

ONGOING EXPANSION

The Touching Hands Project has grown rapidly since 2014. The first annual report was published in 2015. Six missions had been successfully completed, and the report was replete with vignettes and heartwarming stories. The 2018 annual report (https://www.assh.org/touching-hands/About-Us/Annual-Report) outlines the impact with 12 countries visited, 320 volunteers participated, and more than 500 cases performed. The report highlights international and domestic efforts along with independent missions. In 2018, 7 cities participated in domestic outreach.

INTERNATIONAL HAND SURGERY TRAVELING FELLOWSHIP

Frasier Leversedge, MD and Mark Baratz, MD led a campaign to raise money for the Scott H. Kozin International Travelling Fellowship. The purpose of this fund was to provide financial support for an annual award to an individual from a developing country to travel to North America and to visit centers of excellence for a minimum of 4 weeks. The goal was to enhance the awardee's knowledge and expertise in hand surgery. The fellowship experience would culminate with participation at the ASSH Annual Meeting. The selected individual would take this knowledge back to their community to improve hand surgery and rehabilitation.

The fundraising goal was $250,000, and the money was quickly obtained from generous donors. The Scott H. Kozin International Travelling Fellowship was announced at the 2018 Annual Meeting in Boston. The first awardee is Lokraj Chaurasia, MD from Nepal, and his fellowship is slated for 2019. He will travel to North America for 4 weeks to advance his hand and upper limb education. Dr Chaurasia's fellowship will culminate as an attendee at the 2019 ASSH Annual Meeting in Las Vegas.

This fellowship represents a further expansion of the ASSH's commitment to global outreach. The fellowship will be offered on a yearly basis to surgeons from developing countries in need of education, knowledge, and experience in hand surgery.

THE REVERSE COMMUTE

The team members of The Touching Hands Project are talented, devoted, and caring health professionals. The members often work in simple environments devoid of the facilities and amenities offered in the United Sates, such as operating microscope and fluoroscopy. Occasionally, a patient with a complex problem cannot be cared for safely in country. The surgeon should avoid (at all cost) putting the patient and The Touching Hands project in jeopardy.

A collaborative effort between The Touching Hands Project, Shriners Hospitals for Children, and NGOs has resulted in a viable solution for these patients in need (also known as The Reverse Commute). The Touching Hands Project has identified the patient. The NGO has provided transportation, housing, and logistics. Shriners Hospitals for Children has provided free medical care for complex procedures. The relationship has resulted in numerous children being treated for complex conditions who would otherwise never be treated. Procedures have included free tissue transfers to overcome bony deficits secondary to trauma and/or infection, massive burn reconstructions, and other orthopedic nonhand orthopedic conditions that were evaluated during the mission (scoliosis and Rickets with bowed legs).

EFFECTIVENESS OF HAND SURGERY CIRCA 2019

Chung and colleagues[5] have analyzed the cost-effectiveness of humanitarian hand surgery trips to low- and middle-income countries. The Touching Hands Project and the Resurge International hands missions were used to formulate the database. The World Health Organization methodology (WHO-Choosing Interventions That Are Cost-Effective) was used to determine whether the procedures performed during the outreach efforts was cost-effective. The cost-effectiveness was determined by calculating the potential benefit of performing the various procedures using disability-adjusted life-years averted score, and the total cost of the trip. A disability-adjusted life is considered a healthy year lost owing to the morbidity and mortality of a medical or surgical condition. The cost-effectiveness of global hand surgery was comparable to other medical conditions, such as treatment of multidrug-resistant tuberculosis in similar regions. The investigators did find a deficiency in the standardization of record keeping that is currently being rectified to allow uniform collection of data and further data analysis.

FUTURE

Outreach and The Touching Hands Project have been solidly established as part of the ASSH. The first outreach director (Don Lalonde, MD) was elected in 2018 to the council of the ASSH. This position provides a seat at the table for future decisions and directions of the ASSH with the goal mirroring the mission and vision of The Touching Hands Project. The project will continue to provide free hand surgery and hand therapy to adults and children in underserved communities around the world. The volunteers will continue to perform hand surgery, provide hand therapy, teach local doctors, build relationships, and change lives. The ultimate goal is that 1 day all those who suffer from a hand injury or deformity will have access to affordable specialized treatment from caring, compassionate, and highly skilled hand professionals with the added benefit of volunteers receiving life-enriching experiences.

REFERENCES

1. Carter PR. The embryogenesis of the specialty of hand surgery: a story of three great Americans—a politician, a general, and a duck hunter: the 2002 Richard J. Smith memorial lecture. J Hand Surg 2003; 28A:185–98.
2. Kozin SH. The richness of caring for the poor: the development and implementation of the touching hands project. J Hand Surg 2015;40:566–75.
3. Brand PW, Yancey P. The gift of pain. New York: Harper Collins/Zondervan; 1993.
4. Meara JG, Hagander L, Leather AJM. Surgery and global health: a Lancet Commission. Lancet 2014; 383:12–3.
5. Qiu X, Nasser JS, Sue GR, et al. Cost-effectiveness analysis of humanitarian hand surgery trips according to WHO-CHOICE thresholds. J Hand Surg Am 2019; 44:93–103.

UNITED STATES POSTAL SERVICE®

Statement of Ownership, Management, and Circulation
(All Periodicals Publications Except Requester Publications)

1. Publication Title	2. Publication Number	3. Filing Date
HAND CLINICS	000 – 709	9/18/2019

4. Issue Frequency	5. Number of Issues Published Annually	6. Annual Subscription Price
FEB, MAY, AUG, NOV	4	$435.00

7. Complete Mailing Address of Known Office of Publication *(Not printer) (Street, city, county, state, and ZIP+4®)*

ELSEVIER INC.
230 Park Avenue, Suite 800
New York, NY 10169

Contact Person
STEPHEN R. BUSHING

Telephone *(Include area code)*
215-239-3688

8. Complete Mailing Address of Headquarters or General Business Office of Publisher *(Not printer)*

ELSEVIER INC.
230 Park Avenue, Suite 800
New York, NY 10169

9. Full Names and Complete Mailing Addresses of Publisher, Editor, and Managing Editor *(Do not leave blank)*

Publisher *(Name and complete mailing address)*

TAYLOR BALL, ELSEVIER INC.
1600 JOHN F KENNEDY BLVD. SUITE 1800
PHILADELPHIA, PA 19103-2899

Editor *(Name and complete mailing address)*

LAUREN BOYLE, ELSEVIER INC.
1600 JOHN F KENNEDY BLVD. SUITE 1800
PHILADELPHIA, PA 19103-2899

Managing Editor *(Name and complete mailing address)*

PATRICK MANLEY, ELSEVIER INC.
1600 JOHN F KENNEDY BLVD. SUITE 1800
PHILADELPHIA, PA 19103-2899

10. Owner *(Do not leave blank. If the publication is owned by a corporation, give the name and address of the corporation immediately followed by the names and addresses of all stockholders owning or holding 1 percent or more of the total amount of stock. If not owned by a corporation, give the names and addresses of the individual owners. If owned by a partnership or other unincorporated firm, give its name and address as well as those of each individual owner. If the publication is published by a nonprofit organization, give its name and address.)*

Full Name	Complete Mailing Address
WHOLLY OWNED SUBSIDIARY OF REED/ELSEVIER, US HOLDINGS	1600 JOHN F KENNEDY BLVD. SUITE 1800 PHILADELPHIA, PA 19103-2899

11. Known Bondholders, Mortgagees, and Other Security Holders Owning or Holding 1 Percent or More of Total Amount of Bonds, Mortgages, or Other Securities. If none, check box ▶ ☐ None

Full Name	Complete Mailing Address
N/A	

12. Tax Status *(For completion by nonprofit organizations authorized to mail at nonprofit rates) (Check one)*
The purpose, function, and nonprofit status of this organization and the exempt status for federal income tax purposes:
☒ Has Not Changed During Preceding 12 Months
☐ Has Changed During Preceding 12 Months *(Publisher must submit explanation of change with this statement)*

PS Form **3526**, July 2014 *(Page 1 of 4 (see instructions page 4)]* PSN: 7530-01-000-9931   PRIVACY NOTICE: See our privacy policy on www.usps.com.

---

13. Publication Title	14. Issue Date for Circulation Data Below
HAND CLINICS	AUGUST 2019

15. Extent and Nature of Circulation			Average No. Copies Each Issue During Preceding 12 Months	No. Copies of Single Issue Published Nearest to Filing Date
a. Total Number of Copies *(Net press run)*			288	317
b. Paid Circulation (By Mail and Outside the Mail)	(1)	Mailed Outside-County Paid Subscriptions Stated on PS Form 3541 *(Include paid distribution above nominal rate, advertiser's proof copies, and exchange copies)*	161	194
	(2)	Mailed In-County Paid Subscriptions Stated on PS Form 3541 *(Include paid distribution above nominal rate, advertiser's proof copies, and exchange copies)*	0	0
	(3)	Paid Distribution Outside the Mails Including Sales Through Dealers and Carriers, Street Vendors, Counter Sales, and Other Paid Distribution Outside USPS®	75	93
	(4)	Paid Distribution by Other Classes of Mail Through the USPS *(e.g. First-Class Mail®)*	0	0
c. Total Paid Distribution *(Sum of 15b (1), (2), (3), and (4))*		▶	236	287
d. Free or Nominal Rate Distribution (By Mail and Outside the Mail)	(1)	Free or Nominal Rate Outside-County Copies included on PS Form 3541	36	13
	(2)	Free or Nominal Rate In-County Copies Included on PS Form 3541	0	0
	(3)	Free or Nominal Rate Copies Mailed at Other Classes Through the USPS *(e.g. First-Class Mail)*	0	0
	(4)	Free or Nominal Rate Distribution Outside the Mail *(Carriers or other means)*	0	0
e. Total Free or Nominal Rate Distribution *(Sum of 15d (1), (2), (3) and (4))*		▶	36	13
f. Total Distribution *(Sum of 15c and 15e)*		▶	272	300
g. Copies not Distributed *(See instructions to Publishers #4 (page #3))*		▶	16	17
h. Total *(Sum of 15f and g)*		▶	288	317
i. Percent Paid *(15c divided by 15f times 100)*		▶	86.76%	95.67%

* If you are claiming electronic copies, go to line 16 on page 3. If you are not claiming electronic copies, skip to line 17 on page 3.

PS Form **3526**, July 2014 *(Page 2 of 4)*

16. Electronic Copy Circulation	Average No. Copies Each Issue During Preceding 12 Months	No. Copies of Single Issue Published Nearest to Filing Date
a. Paid Electronic Copies ▶		
b. Total Paid Print Copies (Line 15c) + Paid Electronic Copies (Line 16a) ▶		
c. Total Print Distribution (Line 15f) + Paid Electronic Copies (Line 16a) ▶		
d. Percent Paid (Both Print & Electronic Copies) (16b divided by 16c x 100) ▶		

☒ I certify that 50% of all my distributed copies (electronic and print) are paid above a nominal price.

17. Publication of Statement of Ownership

☒ If the publication is a general publication, publication of this statement is required. Will be printed
in the __November 2019__ issue of this publication.   ☐ Publication not required.

18. Signature and Title of Editor, Publisher, Business Manager, or Owner	Date
Stephen R. Bushing	9/18/2019

STEPHEN R. BUSHING - INVENTORY DISTRIBUTION CONTROL MANAGER

I certify that all information furnished on this form is true and complete. I understand that anyone who furnishes false or misleading information on this form or who omits material or information requested on the form may be subject to criminal sanctions (including fines and imprisonment) and/or civil sanctions (including civil penalties).

PS Form **3526**, July 2014 *(Page 3 of 4)*   PRIVACY NOTICE: See our privacy policy on www.usps.com.

Moving?

Make sure your subscription moves with you!

To notify us of your new address, find your **Clinics Account Number** (located on your mailing label above your name), and contact customer service at:

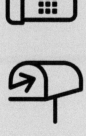

Email: journalscustomerservice-usa@elsevier.com

800-654-2452 (subscribers in the U.S. & Canada)
314-447-8871 (subscribers outside of the U.S. & Canada)

Fax number: 314-447-8029

Elsevier Health Sciences Division
Subscription Customer Service
3251 Riverport Lane
Maryland Heights, MO 63043

*To ensure uninterrupted delivery of your subscription, please notify us at least 4 weeks in advance of move.

ELSEVIER

Printed and bound by CPI Group (UK) Ltd, Croydon, CR0 4YY

03/10/2024

01040371-0010